Supercharged Mom

Takes Back Health & Vitality

12 Steps To Success For Special Needs Families

Copyright © 2016 Lara Franks
All rights reserved.
First published: January, 2017
Printed by: Createspace
ISBN-10: 154136175X
ISBN-13: 978-1541361751

To Larry, Chanchie, Mickle Tickle, Smalls, and Jo:

You are the journey, the reason, the gifts, the inspiration. You are the love and the light that drive my breath and my life. I cannot imagine a minute without you.

CONTENTS

My Journey

I was sitting off to the side at a social gathering chatting to the woman next to me. I knew her socially, and one of her youngsters had worked in one of my businesses through high school. She gazed out at the crowd and suddenly turned to me and said; "My children have been such a disappointment to me." I was floored. I was aware that her children had special needs, but I knew them, and never would have described them that way. They may have had their issues, but they were well-mannered, likable and handsome young people. I gathered my thoughts and responded: "Well, my son has been a real blessing to us. He has taken our family on a journey we would otherwise never have had the opportunity to experience!"

What a journey it has been. We had crossed a continent in search of help for our children and a better quality of life for our family. What we discovered is that the crazy roller coaster ride of life does not slow down, but how you handle the ride makes all the difference.

Life in Southern California seemed idyllic. Family and friends abounded, and the weather was just perfect. Our daughters were born two and one half years apart. I worked through both pregnancies, and returned to work soon after. My oldest daughter was slow to speak. She had her own language, and would babble away happily, a sweet and gentle child. She loved all creatures, from the tiniest ladybug she found in our garden, to the largest horse she could ride at the regional park. She was reluctant to potty train, but we had heard that some kids are, so we hung in there. She went to preschool at the age of three, and we expressed concern to the preschool director about her delayed speech, which was just emerging. Her response to us: "She's a woman, she'll talk", and eventually she did. And life moved on.

Our second daughter was a model baby. She was born sucking her thumb, and instead of crying would soothe herself with it as she settled down for naps and sleep. By the age of eighteen months she was conversing in full sentences. We knew we wanted a big family, so we decided not to wait, and when she was only five months old I got pregnant with number three.

My little prince came barreling out at over eight pounds. One look and I was smitten. He had a laugh that gurgled up from his belly, and a smile that lit up the room. Aside from recurring ear infections coupled with high fevers, he progressed as expected, meeting milestones for crawling, walking, and self-feeding, and constantly laughing at the antics of his sisters. Then suddenly he stalled. Around 18 months, as the other toddlers at Mommy and

Me group started using their words, he was silently playing in the corner. When the other toddlers started sharing and playing together, he played alone. But again, everyone we spoke to delivered the same platitudes: "Boys develop slower than girls, so give it time." By this time I was pregnant with number four, so out of sheer exhaustion I plodded on, even though I sensed something was amiss.

Then the screaming set in. If we took a different route to preschool, he shrieked as if in pain. Try as I might, I could not get him to string three words together. He pulled at certain fabrics against his body, writhing to get out of them. From a baby with a healthy appetite, his diet was reduced to about five foods. He went to preschool, but was in his own world there. Separation from me in the morning was agonizing, and the final straw was him biting a teacher. We were advised to get testing, but it was only conducted by the school district at age three, so we waited for an appointment. I already suspected the diagnosis, and I was right. Autism. The roller coaster ride had just begun, or so we *erroneously* thought. Little did we know at that point that we would be on a journey with more than one child.

Initial reactions: shock, fear, panic, anger, devastation, depression. Scrambling to make sense of it all was overwhelming. He was placed in a county program, and my limited research led me to understand that it was hopelessly inadequate. So afternoons became journeys to private therapists in the hope that double doses of early intervention would speed up his progress. I don't even remember my beautiful baby daughter at that age. I feel like I lost a whole chunk of her life. Those months became a blur as I trekked around from school to therapy, researching late into the night and living in a state of anxiety and sleep-deprivation.

I had wanted a fourth child and had fantasized about how wonderful it would be to have another son, so that everyone could have a sister and a brother. When we received the Autism diagnosis, I called the pediatrician in a panic! He warned us that my adorable six month old son would be 50% at risk of being on the Autism spectrum too. For anyone who has been down this path, you will understand the anxiety of the waiting game. Every developmental move is analyzed, every milestone meticulously charted, every vaccination considered and timed as if to ward off the "evil eye" from sabotaging this precious new life. We passed twelve months. At eighteen months we still held our breaths. By twenty-four months I started to let out some air, and by three years old we knew we were in the clear. My autistic son would have a baby brother who was neuro-typical, and hopefully a best friend!

Meanwhile, during this period I was clashing with the school district, who in their infinite wisdom had decided to teach my older son sign language, instead of how to speak. A well-meaning social worker from the county informed me that I should expect that there was an 85% chance he would be mentally retarded, that he would probably never speak, or have a meaningful relationship with another person, be able to drive a car, or handle money, and the list went on. By the time she was finished with me I had decided that that would *never* be my child. Back online I went looking for options. I came across a wonderful center for Autism in Baltimore, and after an exploratory trip, we packed up our children and headed east to find help and maybe regain some sanity.

Remember my earlier comment about the roller coaster? Well the ride sure does not end. In our new town, my daughters were enrolled in a private school, and my son was placed in an Autism program through the IEP process - an Individual Education Plan (more on that later). With a fifteen month old on my hip, I now drove two carpools in the morning, then picked him up at lunch, and started on the private Speech Language Therapy and Occupational Therapy circuit in the afternoons, then back to grab the girls and head home. I hired afternoon and evening help to deal with the boys while I threw macaroni or fish sticks together for dinner, and helped the girls with homework.

Then other problems arose. My oldest daughter was being bullied, and was experiencing difficulties with social relationships and friendships. Her manner of verbal expression was still a little out of the ordinary, and we were working with enough therapists for me to feel instinctively that something was amiss. I decided to have her tested and ADHD was the diagnosis. Well, I felt like a real failure. Had I been so wrapped up with my son that I had totally missed the signs? Missing out on my younger daughter's toddlerhood, and now subjecting my new baby to a toddlerhood spent in the waiting rooms of various therapists, instead of at Mommy and Me classes, or naps in his crib. What was I doing to my family? I sank into a dark place, lying unresponsive on the couch, not wanting to go on with this life. My shocked husband put all four children in the car, loaded me in, and took me to a therapist. It was my first and only experience with a mental health professional, but she managed to get me to acknowledge that I was doing all I could do, and I needed to plod forward without trying to be Supermom.

And so I did. Helping my husband in his business, juggling four young children, two with special needs and accommodations, and forgetting myself in the process, was how life rolled on. Spending time on my marriage was definitely not a priority. I was lucky to just be getting through the day on large amounts of caffeine, diet soda, and whatever food I could eat while driving, or sitting in a waiting room, or picking off my kids plates. Cooking – very rarely. Sleep – ha, totally overrated anyway. A gym – well, wasn't that a big room located somewhere inside a school building. Exercise – ever tried running behind a non-verbal, three and a half year old Autistic boy whose only goal is to run anywhere he can get to, while lugging a nice chubby fifteen month old on your hip? Friendships – luckily we had a Sabbath, and made sure to use it to make plans with other families in order to maintain a social circle. And so my life limped on, solely focused on the children and their needs, my husband's and my needs relegated to a back burner.

When my youngest son was in second grade, the school experienced some unusual instability with staffing, and he landed up having 5 teachers in 1 year. I was deeply concerned that the class had lost a year of instruction, and we transferred him to the school we had moved my older daughter to, in order to extract her from a negative social dynamic. As the year started, I received a call from the Vice Principal, who case managed the students with learning differences. The teachers reported that my youngest was very restless in class, and was not meeting benchmarks for reading and reading comprehension. He was also struggling to write. Testing was recommended, and he was diagnosed with acute ADD and dysgraphia. It turned out we were three for four in our house, and things were only going to get more complicated!

Just as life seemed as if it could not possibly get crazier, there were new challenges and surprises around each bend. The turning point arrived in the form of a visit from my brother. He stood in the kitchen watching me go through the witching hours from 4:00 to 7:00 p.m. each evening, relying on copious amounts of caffeine and diet soda to keep me running, and shoveling anything within reach into my mouth as dinner. I then ended each evening with a blinding headache. He vocalized most emphatically that this was a recipe for disaster, and made me promise that after he left I would try and eliminate the caffeine and artificial sweeteners from my diet. I gave it a go, and lo and behold, the headaches subsided dramatically. I had already started working out regularly, and knew I wanted to learn more about how to feel healthier. I was still tired, not getting enough sleep, constantly stressed and short on time, and about twenty-five pounds overweight. I look back in great sadness when I see how few family photos I allowed myself to be in due to embarrassment about my weight!

I started reading books about improving one's health, and all the incremental changes I made in diet and lifestyle made a significant difference. During one of my online searches I found the Institute for Integrative Nutrition®, or IIN®. I realized there and then that I wanted to focus on the links between nutrition and good health, and share it with as many people as I could, beginning with my own family. Enrolling in the Health Coach Training Program changed my life and the lives of my family for the better. It is hard to imagine how, as a mother already juggling a job, children with so many special needs, financial stresses, and time constraints, that you can ever climb out of that rut. I am here to tell you that it is possible. In addition, when you improve the quality of your own health and well-being, and then implement simple strategies to improve the lives of your family, life actually becomes *easier*. The other powerful benefit is that you create longevity. A huge cause of concern and stress for parents of significantly impaired children is what will become of them if and when a parent passes away. By confronting how you take care of yourself, and by making incremental improvements (even if the process is slow and daunting), you have taken the first steps to mitigating whatever may undermine your own health.

A journey of life, through the challenges of bringing up children with learning differences and special needs, automatically starts to exclude the extraneous. There is only time to focus on getting through the basics and essentials of daily living, coupled with work and the children's services. The road is paved with potholes, setbacks, stress, a lot of pain and tears. As parents, we grasp onto every moment of laughter, joy, success, and peace that bursts through. There is no time or thought for keeping up appearances, driving the latest model car or having the nicest house. Perfect, high achieving kids are not part of our lexicon. Trotting out the latest fashions or having a weekly manicure is for people who live in an alternate universe.

I would never trade my experiences for any of those things. On my journey, I have learned who I am, what I am capable of feeling, my levels of strength and resilience, the depths of my love for my husband and my children, and a debt of gratitude to our parents that I know I could never repay. When life punches you and your family in the gut, you learn how to come back stronger. You certainly come to understand really fast who is on your team - those who are cheering you on from the sidelines.

As I began to write this book, I remembered something I had read years before. In *The Child with Special Needs* by Stanley I. Greenspan, M.D., he cautions parents about "… throwing themselves into a quest to obtain the best possible help from specialists, leaving little of themselves for daily nurturing."[1] As parents, we need to nurture and support ourselves emotionally, spiritually and physically in order to cope with the demands of our journey and to be present for our children in all of those capacities.

This book is about how I came back stronger and healthier, against the odds, to lead my family though a transformation to health and vitality. The chapters that follow are in order of the steps I took in my journey, but others might choose a different path to health, and that is perfectly fine. I hope that some of my strategies will be useful tools for you to integrate into your own life, or, at the very least, to empower you to chart your own course into healing and self-discovery. Read it in sequence, or open to the chapter that speaks most urgently to you. Adopt one tip, or try to phase in a few. It does not really matter. What is important is that this is about our unique journeys, and the small steps we take to cope better while on it will yield tremendous benefits for our well-being and that of our families. You owe it to yourself and your children, so please take the first step with me.

---

[1] Greenspan, Stanley, *The Child With Special Needs* (Perseus Books, 1998)

Part One — The Why:

BUILDING YOUR INNER STRENGTH

Your Inner Voice

After my son was diagnosed with Autism, I started looking into various therapies. ABA (Applied Behavior Analysis) was just starting to become one of the more popular techniques in dealing with non-verbal, autistic children. I watched the videos and researched their practices. I was desperate to get my three-and-a-half year old to string a few simple words together so I could just meet his most basic needs of "I'm hungry" or "I'm thirsty." There is nothing more frightening than having your child be unable to communicate his basic needs to you. The ABA therapy would cost a small fortune, but I would have paid it. Yet, something inside me did not feel right. Maybe I was just not ready to acknowledge that I had a child who needed something so severe in its practices. I was feeling emotionally fragile, and was not sure I could withstand the hours of endless screaming I knew would ensue, or to watch my son be forced through a routine time and time again until he complied with a single instruction.

Instead, I opted to find a really good speech language pathologist. It was the right decision for my son. Speech language pathology has a totally different approach, and he blossomed. In retrospect, it was this seemingly small decision — to listen to my gut — that spelled the difference between a happy and successful path forward versus what might have been a painful and constraining path of setbacks and frustration for my son.

Another example of trusting my inner voice arose soon after moving to Baltimore and enrolling my son in an Autism program in a county school. He started behaving peculiarly when I would walk him towards his classroom. He would cover his eyes, and try and run for the front door. I sensed that something was not right. I approached the teacher after school as soon as I could catch her, and inquired as to how things were going. She told me that my (non-verbal) child was not very compliant, and that he often had to spend time in the time-out chair. I also discovered that she was rough when physically handling him. I immediately pulled him from the school, even though it meant he was home and not receiving vital services, until we could arrange an alternative placement for him.

As parents, we have *built-in instincts*. When your inner voice starts complaining that something feels off, it probably *is*. When you leave an IEP Team meeting questioning why the word "team" is used in that context, it is time to take action. When your pediatrician tells you that changing your child's diet won't help their asthma or eczema and that medication is your only solution, yet every time you serve a dairy meal their symptoms worsen, do your own research. If your child tells you they are being bullied at school, and the school tells you there is no evidence to support that, do your homework (siblings and other kids make great spies!).

Your inner voice is more than just a conscience. It is an *alarm* and a *thermostat*. It sounds a warning that all is not well, or that situations need to be modified or improved. Keep a journal next to your bed. At night, write down what your inner voice told you that day. Track these messages and see what patterns develop. Sometimes it will turn out to be a fleeting feeling about something that happened that may never reoccur. If that is the case, you are probably safe letting it go. However, your inner voice may be yelling out to you with some frequency that something does not seem right. If you see a pattern emerge, chances are good there is some legitimacy there and you need to address it.

Part of trusting your inner voice requires focusing on *modulating that voice.* You have to learn how to be your child's champion because no one else is going to care as deeply for his or her well-being and success. When a doctor, therapist, or teacher tells you one thing, and you whole-heartedly believe another, you have to modulate your inner voice into the warrior or the drill sergeant, and fight it out until you have a resolution you can live with. If I had listened to the school in California, my son would have been most adept at sign language but not be able to speak! You also have to develop tenacity, and that is not easy. You may be afraid that people are going to think you are pushy, rude, disrespectful, or even someone to be avoided at all costs. I will let you in on a little secret. I have never been comfortable embracing tenacity, but allowing it to be the expression of my inner voice at critical junctures has been perhaps the single most valuable tool in my "Coping Mom" toolbox.

Be heard. Don't let the voices of others drown out your inner voice. It could be a domineering spouse or parent, it could be a friend whose feelings you do not want to hurt. It could be a pediatrician who asserts that *they* are the medical professional, and they discourage us laymen and women from offering our opinions. No matter how loud someone else is screaming about what you should do with regard to your child, give voice to your inner thoughts, feelings and intuitions, and come back louder. Your child's well-being is at stake!

You may be wondering what this has to do with ultimate health and vitality. Your inner voice is not just a hunch about something. It can also literally be a voice expressing your thoughts and feelings in a very real way. When you give voice to those thoughts and feelings, it can be very liberating, and in some cases highly therapeutic and healing. Years later, after we withdrew my son from the private school in which he was bullied, I found I still held a lot of pent up anger inside my soul. I was mostly angry at the principal of the middle school, who first denied the accusations, then dismissed the incidents as "horseplay," and then after witnesses saw my son being attacked, chose not to hold anyone accountable. An opportunity arose two years later when I encountered him alone in a store. I thought to myself "it's now or never!" I walked right up to him and told him how much pain he had caused our family through the way he had dealt with the situation. I felt liberated at finally being able to articulate what had been festering inside me for so long. Now when I see him I just look through him. He does not bother me anymore. I exorcized that negativity from my body and my life and I feel so much better for it!

I am not sure that we appreciate how much negativity we keep pent up inside our bodies and our souls while on this journey. Emotional health is an extensive subject and beyond the scope of this book. Suffice to say that you cannot achieve health and vitality without addressing your emotional state. I have a special word that I feel encapsulates it for me: *Resilience.* Resilience means the ability to bounce back from adversity. It suggests a certain toughness, thick skin, and broad shoulders on which to bear your load. Often all that is required to accomplish this is a mental attitude adjustment, a way in which to view our circumstances through a new lens, from a new perspective, a viewpoint that strengthens us rather than weakening us. However, for many parents it may require the help and support of a mental health professional, a social worker, or an experienced health coach. I am confident that if you begin the process by not negating your inner voice, but by giving credence to it and believing in your own inner strength and parental instincts, you will ultimately be successful in overcoming what may now seem emotionally overwhelming. You will certainly have a better sense of what the primary drivers of your emotions are. If you listen carefully, I think you will also hear your inner voice directing you regarding whether you are able to work through the challenge by yourself, or whether it is time to call in the professional reinforcement!

I want to touch briefly here on advocacy, which bears a more detailed discussion in the next chapter. I receive calls from many parents who are referred to me by teachers, friends, and an organization I serve on the Board of, which provides services to special needs children. During the writing of this very chapter, a mother called to seek my opinion. It was recommended to her by a private therapist that her daughter receive a speech language evaluation in addition to psycho-educational testing. The school district, which was mandated to provide the free testing, did not feel the speech language tests were necessary. This mother did not know what to do. It was her first encounter with the IEP process. I recommended that she fight for a complete set of tests. Without a complete picture of the child, how could parents and teachers be sure what problem areas need to be addressed in an educational plan? Listen to your inner voice, be confident in its messages, and take action for the sake of your child and your family. (An explanation of the IEP process can be found in the following chapter.)

TUNE IN:

As a first step, practice tuning in and listening to your inner voice.

Do not analyze the meaning. Simply practice gathering the data from the far reaches of your mind.

MY INNER VOICE SAYS ...	IT IS RESPONDING TO...

SUCCESS STEP TWO:

Building Your Team

It most definitely takes a village to successfully navigate a life made up of multiple facets that could include relationships or marriage, special needs children, parenting their non-disabled, neuro-typical siblings, holding a job, running a home, maintaining relationships with family and friends, and simply navigating the maze of daily living. The goal here is for mom and dad to maintain optimal health in order to achieve longevity, as well as finding that daily vitality that makes an enormous difference when managing all of the above, while still being your child's most powerful advocate. Phew! This is a tall order, and without a supportive network, the burden falls solely on the primary caregiver, which more often than not means the mother.

Many mothers get the first half of the equation right, the part about doing for others and seeing to their needs, and the daily demands of life. The second part not so much. I speak from the perspective of being one of those moms. The years of self-sacrifice are long, and for some there appears to be no end in sight. Many mothers lose sight of themselves on this journey. Once vibrant, often highly educated and professionally proficient young women with hopes and dreams of bright futures, may find themselves trapped in a world they could not have imagined or conceived of in their younger days. There is only one way back from this. You have to develop a team. If you are to loosen the chains and begin to recover yourself, someone else it going to have to pick up the slack. It is not a choice. It is a necessity. Being the best that you can be means you have the opportunity to give the best that you can give, and who would *not* want that power?

Building a team means surrounding yourself with people who not only provide emotional support, but also professionals who provide valued therapies and medical interventions, and most importantly, folks who can provide respite. One mother I interviewed, let's call her Deidre, shared that even before her son was formally diagnosed with Asperger's, her friends, who were like her family, were incredibly sensitive to her situation, while at the same time giving her gentle, non-threatening words of advice about what to do with her non-typically developing child. After his diagnosis, they became his greatest advocates, which provided Deidre and her family with tremendous love and emotional support. Her support group helped remove the stigma of his diagnosis by fully embracing her family. My son has the same diagnosis, and it was so interesting to compare notes and realize that both of us had coped so well because of our shared experience of having strong teams at our sides, while at the same time realizing that not everyone is as successful at creating this network.

My son is a few years younger than hers, and she mentioned something I had actually given no thought to. When our children are younger, we try to surround them with peers who can role model age-typical behaviors. Many special needs children are in some form of an inclusion environment to this same end. However, as the years go by and special needs children graduate high school, their non-disabled "friends" and classmates progress to the point where there is no longer social engagement. Now parents are faced with a different challenge - how to assist their young adults in forming a social circle in order to prevent isolation and depression. In the case of Diedre, the young adults in her circle continue to engage her son intermittently, but as they marry and establish family lives, that time will dwindle. Diedre now has to build a different team, or widen her circle. She has to seek out families with other impacted young adults and find opportunities to develop friendships between these young men and women. It is a constant work-in-progress, necessitating a willingness to remain open-minded and aware, connected and ready to make connections, while at the same time vigilantly evaluating the quality of these relationships.

It is necessary to use a set of criteria to evaluate who best fits your team in order to avoid becoming embroiled in toxic relationships that do not serve you well. Based on your personality, try to establish which qualities are important in the individuals who will be supporting you and your child on your journey. Be honest.

Know what *your* needs are when it comes to . . .

Family and Friends:

Are you ok with freely given advice, or do you want to be the initiator?

Would you be comfortable with them sharing your child's diagnosis and challenges, or would you prefer that they maintain your privacy?

Do you want the casseroles and the carpools, or do you need someone who has time for a girls' night out and a good glass of wine?

Should your friends be good for a few laughs, or is it more valuable for them to be a great shoulder to cry on?

Professionals:

Do you need someone who will soften each blow, or would you function more productively with a straight shooter?

Is it important to you that the members on your team are open-minded and progressive, or does old school traditional make you feel more secure and confident?

Are you able to stand up to an "expert" if your gut strongly disagrees with their professional diagnosis?

Are you drawn to the person with the worldview that the glass is half full or half empty?

Would you prefer to deal with a man or a woman?

All of these are important questions to consider, and the answers will ultimately help shape a team that best inspires your confidence or best provides you with the help and comfort you need. Your criteria will also be pivotal in deciding which therapists and doctors are your child's best advocates.

Your team is essential for your emotional health and well-being. Just knowing that you are loved, accepted and supported on your journey can relieve some of the pain to which we can all succumb at times. When my husband and I decided to move to the East Coast, we consulted with a religious advisor. We wanted to be sure that moving away from our parents and siblings was in fact the appropriate course of action for our family. Our primary reason was to seek a higher quality of services and care for our son. Our secondary reason was to extract ourselves from the daily deluge of family advice and interference in how we were dealing with him. This spiritual counselor said something that could have been profoundly damaging to the creation of our team in our new home, had we listened to him. He cautioned us not to discuss our son's diagnosis publicly in the event that he or our family became stigmatized. Because it was plain for all to see that my child was different, this was impossible. But *because* it was plain to see, people responded to him and reached out to us, sharing their own stories and journeys. Along with that came the sharing of resources, and this really helped us in shaping our team. The best resources are other parents of special needs children who are willing to share their successes and their pitfalls. Oftentimes they also become your best friends, as we have been blessed to experience.

Respite is something that is equally essential for your emotional and physical well-being. It is, however, impossible without team members who are willing to provide it. If you have been successful in receiving state, county or city services that include respite, you are ahead of the game provided you actually take full advantage of these resources. If your child has qualified under an Autism Waiver, that may be part of the package too. However, I know from my own experience that there are many more parents who do not have access to formal respite services, and they have to engineer them on their own. In my case we had two sets of parents (and siblings) within minutes of our home during our California years. All were willing to babysit so that we could have an evening off, or even a night or two away, which was invaluable. A word of caution in this instance, however. No matter how much time your parents spend with your children, they do not *live* with them. They may not truly understand the complexity of the rituals, the nuances of the sensory accommodations, the minuscule catalysts for an emotional explosion, and the necessity of adhering strictly to the established routine. Make sure you prepare them as thoroughly as you can. I recommend creating a mini booklet, just a page or two, maybe inserting an endearing picture. This is a great way to give grandma and grandpa (or any willing babysitter) the lowdown on exactly what they might expect, and especially which buttons to definitely avoid pushing. I did not think to do this, and the following incident unfolded in my house.

My father graciously agreed to babysit one evening. My Aspie boy was about three and a half at the time. I made sure to put all four children to bed and then we headed out. We got home to find my dad in a terrible state. He told us that he had almost gone into cardiac arrest and was really frazzled. Of course we were terribly alarmed. What could have gone so wrong? "Well, I thought I had lost your son!" said my quadruple-bypass-I-don't-have-the-strongest-ticker dad! He proceeded to relate the story.

All was quiet upstairs, but he went up anyway to peek at the children. He discovered my son's bed was empty. He figured maybe he had wandered into my bed, so he went to look. Our room was empty. He went to check if he had crawled in with one of his sisters. Nope, they were sleeping peacefully and the baby was in his crib, alone! Now my father was starting to worry, but he figured an Asperger's child is different so maybe he preferred the bathtub. Checked both bathtubs for a sleeping child – nothing.

Now really bad stuff started going through my dad's head. It was not so long ago that a small child was abducted through the window of her bedroom. He checked all the windows, but they were locked tight. He had been reading in the living room at the base of the staircase and he knew for a fact that my son had not come down. I wish in retrospect that he had just called us at that point, but being the selfless, generous man that he is, he really wanted us to have an uninterrupted evening. He stood on the landing upstairs not knowing how he was going to tell us when we got home that he had literally lost our precious son. Suddenly, out of the corner of his eye, he spied the couch on the large landing that we used as an upstairs play area. It appeared to be empty, but my dad was leaving no stone (or in this case, pillow) unturned. Lo and behold, my son had burrowed all the way down the back of the couch, under all of the cushions and throw pillows, and was sleeping peacefully. We had forgotten to tell our parents a really important detail: my son craved deep pressure when he went to sleep. It calmed his nervous system. He would pull all of his pillows and blankets onto his body at night to weigh him down. He was obviously seeking that pressure, and burrowing into the couch provided it. Had I thought to make that little booklet for babysitters all those years back, it would have saved my father the undue anxiety he had experienced!

I did, however, make that booklet for the classroom teachers at the beginning of each school year throughout elementary school, and even for my son's transition to sixth grade. It had a cover page with a cute picture of him and one additional "All about Me" page. This leads us into the discussion of parental advocacy, your school team, and the broader question: Is your IEP team really on *your* team?

This book is about learning how to achieve a modicum of emotional well-being, and this is a challenge when every step over the threshold of your child's school unleashes a sizable tremor in your gut that rivals the San Andreas fault on a bad day! Maybe I can dispel some myths right up front by relating a simple request from a good friend of mine who is an IEP Chair at a local high school. I asked him "What can parents do to help foster a positive relationship with their IEP team?" His answer was simple: "Be confident!" I asked him to explain what that meant. He felt that parents needed to come into the process with confidence, having already clearly defined what they are requesting, and having a sense of what challenges they want addressed. If you have not had any formal testing, make a note of examples of deficits or behaviors that are troubling to you. My friend feels that we would serve our children more effectively if we placed a heavier burden on the team to *disprove* our theories about our children or their placements. This sounds crazy, but what he was in fact saying was that things can become very drawn out and contentious when parents walk into a meeting with a feeling that something is off, and then ask the team to help solve an unknown problem. As parents we tend to expect that the team are the problem solvers, when in fact it is *we* who should come to the process prepared to advocate with some facts in hand. That is why testing is done in advance of these meetings, to give both sides time to be adequately prepared. It is incumbent upon us parents to do our due diligence. Research your child's symptoms; discuss them with a pediatrician; maybe pay for private testing if it is within your means. Even if you were not able to have testing in-hand, come to the process educated and prepared to discuss and debate from a position of strength and mutual respect. If you want to close doors, come in yelling and demanding!

If your child already has a plan in place and you are preparing for an upcoming meeting, take a printed copy of the proposed IEP with you. Highlight your concerns in one color. Highlight words or paragraphs on which you need further clarification in another color. Type out your questions in detail. Make sure that you do not leave the table until you have satisfactory answers. (Just to be clear, these may not always be the answers you are wanting to hear!) Everyone's time is valuable, so make good use of it.

Let us now discuss the IEP team and the process. This team is a collaboration between parents and the local school district. Together they endeavor to prepare an appropriate blueprint for successfully educating a special needs or learning impaired child in the least restrictive setting. The goal is to ensure that the child can be educated, but can do so in an environment that is as close to full inclusion as possible. The team is most commonly comprised of the parents or legal guardian, the IEP Chairperson at the zoned school, a special educator, a general educator, a therapist (one or more of the following: psychologist, guidance counselor, occupational therapist, physical therapist, audiologist, speech language pathologist), and a case manager if the child has one. The school district is mandated, *by law*, to provide a battery of testing when a child enters this process. Thereafter the child is re-assessed at least every three years (in most cases). On receipt of the test results, an IEP meeting is scheduled. At that meeting the team outlines what they perceive to be an appropriate educational plan for your child. This plan will include, where necessary, special accommodations, classroom placement, adaptive services, extended year services (to maintain present levels of academic proficiency), therapies and behavioral interventions (for example social skills groups or a number of hours per month with the school social worker or counselor). Specific goals are set at this meeting, and the child is expected to reach certain benchmarks each semester. At the end of the year the team reconvenes to evaluate the child's performance, and adjusts the plan accordingly for the next school year.

This sounds pretty logical and straightforward, right? Well, it is not! The goals and benchmarks are often incomprehensible or problematic from a parent's perspective. Parents spend inordinately more time with their children and there are often overriding issues we want to see addressed. The school will push back, saying that their only responsibility is to address deficits or behaviors as far as they relate to classroom and academic progress. My feeling is that universal behaviors that impact a child to the point that progress is impeded should be part of the team's focus so that we all address them daily, whether at home or at school. This will maximize our ability to positively affect the child's development. Over the years I have had to be extremely forceful in helping to shape the goals and benchmarks to that end. My tenacity certainly helped to ensure victory in most instances. Let me share an example from my son's IEP in his fourth grade year. He had several gastrointestinal issues as a young child. He would experience frequent bouts of constipation and would become afraid of eliminating because it was painful and uncomfortable. As a result, he had to be carefully managed in order to avoid a critical situation. I wanted the school to be as vigilant as I was being at home. After having to force the issue, the following goal made it onto his IEP:

Social Emotional Goal: Body Elimination

Goal: He will increase his ability to eliminate in the school setting from 0 times a day to 1 time per day during school hours as measured by observation record.

Objective 1: Given instruction and support, he will recognize psycho-social and environmental factors which impact on his elimination patterns

Objective 2: Given instruction and support, he will identify 1-3 ways his elimination problem interferes with school activities

Bingo!

I appreciate that it is not always that simple. I will also admit that, after I withdrew my son from the public school in which he was being hurt physically and emotionally, I was such a mess that we retained the services of a special education attorney. We have had Mark on retainer for many years. It has been the best money we ever spent! As a working mother of four very young children, three with challenges, I was too exhausted and frazzled to dispassionately represent my child. With each change of placement from elementary, to middle, to high school, Mark was there to facilitate our wishes. He attended every year-end IEP team meeting through elementary and middle school to ensure that the services we deemed essential would not be cut, going into the next school year. But more than that, he kept us calm which helped maintain our sanity, and he kept the team meetings cordial and respectful, which helped maintain our relationships with the school staff.

While retaining an attorney is costly, there are other places parents can turn to find team members. In many cities there are non-profit organizations that provide parent advocates free of charge. When we were exploring moving back East, I flew out to visit schools. A local non-profit, referred to me by a friend who is a speech language pathologist, assigned me a parent advocate. She loaded me into her van and drove me around the city to visit private and non-public schools. In addition, she gave me the lay of the land in dealing with the public school system in the neighborhood. I felt like I had a bird's eye view of our options and this was very empowering.

The most powerful team, however, is that of the parents. Your spouse or partner is the one person who has the ability to have your back, and you theirs. That will not happen unless you are both on the same page when making vital decisions that affect the lives of your children. Building consensus between yourselves is critical. It is likely that you may both have differing opinions about services, therapists, or even school placements. It is essential that you each give voice to your opinions, are both heard, and then establish a mutually agreed upon system of evaluation in order to come to a decision. In our marriage, we discuss at length our gut feelings. We then agree to separate our emotions from the facts. Then comes a list of pros and cons of the options that face us. More often than not, we come to a mutually agreeable decision through this process. Sometimes, though, my husband will defer to me since I am the partner who handles most of the school-parent or parent-therapist communication, and who spends more hours per day with the children.

Other ways one can develop invaluable relationships is by attending support groups. As mentioned above, other parents are the greatest source of love, support, friendship, and resources for everything from therapists and schools to mother's helpers and babysitters. My husband and I have not regularly attended support groups. However, the fact that almost all of our closest friends have children with some kind of issue or another constitutes an informal one. This has several powerful implications in our lives. We are able to talk and laugh and cry together as we share stories about our journeys. We feel comfortable enough to share the good, the bad and the ugly, and we know that we can do so safely in the confines of non-judgmental relationships. And most importantly, we can clearly internalize the fact that it is not only our children but our lives as well that are impacted. My husband will often lament in exasperation that our kids are screen addicted, or spoilt, or ungrateful about such and such, as if this did not occur in other people's homes. I feel so vindicated when one of our friends pops up with a similar story, and he then has to admit that it is not just our children who are not perfect, and not just the two of us who feel that our parenting skills are sometimes lacking!

The bottom line is this: Help can be found everywhere. Build your team!

YOUR TEAM:

Outline who your team needs to include to fully support you on your journey. The list may include active team members, as well as members still needing to be recruited.

Team Member	Role In Supporting Me	Where I Will Find Them?

Part Two — The What:
THE MIND/BODY CONNECTION

THE MIND-BODY CONNECTION

Understanding the long-term effects of stress, sleep deprivation and bad habits on your body and your health will become the catalyst to clean up and clean out. Through the years, I had suffered from headaches, stomach aches, inability to lose weight, constant congestion and sinus infections, moodiness, lack of energy, and exhaustion. As I began to understand the link between life-style, nutrition, and these symptoms, I was able to begin the process of eradicating them from my life. It is a process, and I continue to work on it daily. I have yet to master all the battles. One of the primary motivations behind writing this book was the shock I experienced when seeing my lab results after years of pursuing my own optimal health. As good as I thought I was being in controlling my diet, my cholesterol numbers were still not where I wanted them to be. I realized at that point how our lack of x-ray vision into the interior of our bodies precludes us from a full understanding of the results of our efforts. Oftentimes, we see the external benefits and results, like the loss of a few pounds, or the increase in energy. At that point we may be tempted to relax our efforts, thinking that we have made great strides. However, my recommendations are to test and then retest, in order to really evaluate those truths. I had to face the ultimate truth that until I curbed my sugar intake, I was not going to get the results I was working towards.

Our bodies were created to heal themselves. In order for healing to take place, the body has to be purged of any obstacles to this process. Thereafter, in order for the battle to be successful, we have to replenish our internal systems, and provide them with the ammunition they need. Fortification can be in the form of the foods we eat, fluids we drink, supplements we take, and life-style and behavior choices we make. As sophisticated as Western medicine has become, we should not lose sight of the fact that our individual healing may be largely within our own control. Physicians constantly bemoan the fact that, if their patients were less neglectful of their bodies, many of them would not require medical attention at all. Type 2 Diabetes, for example, has been informally termed a life-style disease, as more often than not, patients' life-style choices prompt the onset, just as their choices can in many instances reverse it.

The following topics include some of the issues that have impacted my life. The recommendations I suggest have been helpful in assisting me to overcome them. Please appreciate that each of these subheadings is the subject of many books and large quantities of research. There is so much to say on each topic. My goal is simply to give you enough information to be able to determine which category plays an important role in your health, and warrants more independent research and exploration.

SUCCESS STEP THREE:

Sleep

You have surely heard that a good night's sleep is important, and as parents, we are often focused on the number of hours our children get each night. However, what I don't think parents really appreciate is how a lack of quality sleep can be our greatest undoing. In my earlier years I would get by on five hours a night. I was only really able to get my work contracts and correspondence done after putting my children to bed. I felt I had no choice but to live on caffeine to fire my brain cells during the day. I did not understand the role lack of sleep played in my inability to lose weight, balance my hormones, regulate my moods and combat my cravings until I started reading studies related to sleep and health.

Several of the parents I interviewed while writing this book expressed acute sleep deprivation as one of the overriding consequences of their children's diagnosis, especially in the early years. As an example, a couple of families had infants and toddlers who were fed through nasogastric tubes (ng-tubes) or gastrostomy tubes (g-tubes). Managing tube feeding in youngsters with a diagnosis on top of everything else is mind-numbingly exhausting, and often takes place throughout the night.

The consequences of being subjected to extended periods of lack of sleep are dire. Some of the issues I discovered during my journey that were integral to addressing my own health are as follows:

1. Hormonal Imbalance: When my journey to take back my health started I made two important new friends: leptin and ghrelin. These are two of the many hormones in your body. Leptin says: "Thank you for feeding me! I'm happy and satisfied." Ghrelin says: "Grrrrrr … I'm hungry! Feed me!" He is very demanding! We want leptin to be in the driver's seat or we will fight the weight loss battle and lose. One of the ways we can increase leptin and decrease ghrelin is through sleep. Being tired increases our ghrelin. A good night's sleep increases our leptin. Did you ever notice that you are hungrier when you are tired? Research shows that our appetites increase roughly 25% when we are tired. Another important hormone that is disrupted by lack of sleep is cortisol. Poor sleep habits increase cortisol levels, which induces an inflammatory response in the body. We will touch on this later in more detail. Suffice it to say that while sleeping, your body releases restorative hormones, and when this process is disrupted by poor sleeping habits it can place you at higher risk for obesity, heart disease, and a

compromised immune system. This, in turn, can lead to a multitude of chronic illnesses.

2. Cognitive Impairment: Your impulse responses and reflexes are dulled by lack of sleep, and you are therefore at a higher risk of being in an accident - or even causing one! In addition, your ability to be reasonable and to think clearly in any given situation is diminished.

3. Mood Swings: It takes very little to provoke an already overworked and overwhelmed parent. We are much more likely to lose our patience and our tempers when we suffer from sleep deprivation. This can also induce a rolling tide of negative emotions including irritability, anxiety, anger, depression, and apathy. How often do you find yourself verbally lashing out at your child or your spouse, and then having to try to take back your words with the "I'm sorry, I'm just so tired" excuse?

There are many beneficial suggestions for getting a better night's sleep. Some of my favorite recommendations to clients, which I have found successful in my own life, include:

Daily exercise: I do cardio exercise three mornings a week, and strength train with yoga and Pilates two mornings a week. On those days I fall asleep faster and stay asleep longer. If I had to exercise in the evenings, I would be wound up and less likely to fall asleep quickly. Some people are able to exercise at night and not have their sleep pattern disrupted, but I am not one of them. Experiment and discover what works best for you.

 Try to create a sleep schedule and follow it as closely as you can, for example, turn out your light at 10:00 p.m. sharp, and set an alarm to wake at 6:00 a.m. the following morning. If I am out late, I adjust my sleep schedule and arrange with my husband to take the early shift with the children so I can get as close to 7-8 hours of sleep as possible. When he is exhausted, I offer to take the early shift. Teamwork!

 Unplug from all electronic screens at least an hour, if not more, before bed. If you need help falling asleep, try reading something that does *not* grab your attention to the point of not wanting to put it down. A pleasurable but not-engaging novel or magazine is recommended. I am an avid reader, and when engrossed in a book I could read through the night, so I have to be very disciplined about putting it aside.

 A hot soak in the tub with a few drops of lavender oil is extremely relaxing at night. Lavender oil has been used for medicinal purposes for hundreds of years, and soaking in it before bed can improve the quality of your sleep. Additionally I keep a sachet next to my bed, and often breathe in the scent several times before turning out the light. You may want to place a drop on your pillow.

 After lights out close your eyes and meditate while breathing in and out slowly and deeply. Don't allow your mind to wander, rather, focus on your breathing and on each of your limbs, allowing them to sink down into the mattress one by one, from your feet to your head. I learned this technique many years ago in college as part of my Theatre Arts training, and it really works. You can also purchase guided relaxation or meditation videos or CDs that can be very instructive in guiding this process. I use *The Holosync Solution* from the Centerpointe Research Institute at www.centerpointe.com. There are many resources to be found on the internet.

 Monitor your food and beverage consumption in the evenings. It goes without saying that you should limit your caffeine intake later in the day, as caffeine is a powerful stimulant. In addition, I would recommend limiting fluids from around 3 hours before you retire if you are one of those folks who wake to make bathrooms runs in the middle of the night. Alcohol can also disrupt sleep patterns, so if you are trying to establish a regular sleep schedule, avoid drinking alcohol. I also caution against eating later in the evening. Feeling bloated or gassy, or experiencing heart burn at bedtime are certainly not conducive to a restful night.

 The power of light: The hormone melatonin plays an integral role in the regulation of the sleep cycle. Its activity is suppressed by the light of day in order to keep us in a state of wakefulness. As darkness falls, so melatonin begins the process of

sleep induction. However, because the system that regulates melatonin reacts to light, it is imperative to always sleep in the dark. Darkness is essential for melatonin's regulation of a normal and restful sleep pattern.

For those parents who have children with disrupted sleep patterns, try some of the environmental changes listed above. White noise machines and night lights may be beneficial and soothing. You can also try natural sleep inducers like melatonin, and foods that contain natural sleep triggers like tryptophan, found in turkey. With young children it is important to establish consistent bedtimes. In some instances you may need to incentivize the children with a behavior modification program that includes a system of earning rewards. Whatever system you employ, do not fall into the trap of motivating children with a sugary prize, such as candy or a trip to the ice cream parlor! Later in the book, when we discuss diet, we will discuss the destructive nature of sugar, and just how addictive it can become.

BEST PRACTICES:

Let's phase in best sleep practices.

PRACTICE	HOW I TRIED IT	DAY/DATE
Exercise		
7-8 Hours		
Avoid Screens		
Hot Bath with Essential Oil, Candles, Music		
Meditation And/Or Breathing Exercises		
Monitor Food & Drink Intake		
Lights Out On Time		

SUPERCHARGED MOM

Overcome Your Cravings

Cravings and emotional eating are the catalysts for poor dietary choices. What do you crave, especially when you are tired? Sugar, caffeine, carbs? Why do you think that is? Are you looking for food to give you a quick energy boost because you are dragging? Do you ever find yourself feeling that the choice is between a Snickers Bar and a valium? I would hazard a guess that it is all of the above.

Cravings are a physiological and emotional response to something that is invariably not good for us. Let's start with the physical. If you power up with a skinny mocha latte with sugar and caffeine in the morning, you are going to give yourself a temporary energy jolt as you fuel your blood sugar. But, as we have all experienced, it comes crashing down late morning and you find yourself on the blood sugar roller coaster. The only way to climb the next hill is to reload, so in go the peanut covered M&M's from the gas station, between the dry cleaners and carpool! Am I talking your language? How about that 4:00 to 6:00 p.m. time zone - or more likely, war zone? If the cookie jar is your new best friend at this time, chances are you are compounding a physiological response to the sugar roller coaster with an emotional "cookie versus valium" struggle, as I was. This may very well indicate an imbalance in your life that has nothing to do with actual food, like the seeming impossibility of having to juggle making dinner, supervising homework, feeding the dogs, and bathing the baby, all within the space of an hour! To start the process of ending this cycle, get in touch with what you are craving that is NOT FOOD. Is it more help, five minute meals, or a distraction for the baby? The only way to successfully address the problem is to have that answer at hand. You need to ascertain whether this behavior is driven by a real cookie addiction, or an emotional response to a situation.

If you discover that you have a legitimate food craving, or addiction, my recommendation is to break this cycle first, and get your blood sugar balanced as quickly as possible. Be forewarned that this is a process that can take anywhere from three days, a week, or months of hard work, depending on how severely you are impacted. A great way to jump-start the process is by doing a detox diet - an elimination diet. Through this process I was able to figure out that sugar was my real vice. It was only after I detoxed myself completely off sugar consumption that I was able to liberate myself from powerful food cravings. We will discuss this in more detail in chapter ten, so feel free to skip ahead if you want that information right away. Many certified health coaches are trained to walk clients through a detox, so don't feel you have to do this alone.

When it comes to compulsive eating as a result of a lack of something in our lives that is not food, the process is more complex. It requires self-examination and introspection to ascertain where you need to be more nourished. It may be that you need a regular massage, a hot yoga class, a best friend, a more emotionally engaged spouse, more hugs, great sex (or just sex!).

A journal is an amazingly inexpensive and powerful tool to use to extricate this data from the far reaches of your mind and soul. It is private, revealing, and cathartic as you clarify what you truly need in order to feel healthier and more whole. Once you are armed with this information, you can make adjustments to incorporate changes into your life. A journal can be the place to not only write down your thoughts and feelings, but also to track what you are eating and drinking each day. You can then go back, and with the help of your useful colored highlighters, start to map out patterns and trends. If the scale won't budge, but you notice that almost every day before carpool you are swinging by the local coffee shop to refuel, you may want to cut out the caffeine-milk-sweetener fix and see if this yields results. If you notice that you feel particularly stressed on Wednesday evenings, and then make the link between that and your husbands tennis game, you may realize that on those evenings it would be useful to find a mother's helper instead of going it alone with the children and dinner preparation. Sometimes, when we are forced to take a few minutes to evaluate the rhythm of our lives in black and white, we are shocked at the picture that emerges before us. How, we wonder, did we not notice or make the links between such an obvious pattern of behavior and its effect on our well-being? The answer is quite simple. How often do we, as parents of special needs children, afford ourselves the luxury of focusing so intently on our own lives or needs? Can we get past the guilt that we are self-indulgent even to start this process? I challenge you to try! Bear in mind that, armed with your valuable new journal data, you can also engage the help of a coach or therapist to create a set of steps on which to climb out of your untenable situation.

CRAVING TRIGGERS:

Try a simple table, like the example below, to track the triggers to your cravings, and document your responses.

DAY & TIME	CRAVING FOR	TRIGGER	HOW AM I FEELING?	MY ACTION PLAN

Find Your Energy

Most people find themselves needing a "pick-me-up" at some point during the day. How much more so do we, the parents tending to the needs of special children, require something to rev up our engines? However, beware of falling prey to the craving crashing roller coasters, especially those induced by the first morning java chip latte and bagel from the drive through, between school, work, therapy, and the grocery store. Being inadequately fueled, or fueled with inferior quality "gas", can make the difference between getting through the day with an upbeat sense of vitality, or barely hanging on. I have learned some valuable lessons on keeping my energy up, and they are the following:

Lesson One – Sleep

Restorative deep sleep, as discussed in Success Step Three, is of primary importance to maintaining energy throughout the day.

Lesson Two – Hydrate

Up to seventy-five percent of Americans walk around daily in a chronically dehydrated state. Somehow, the notion that drinking eight glasses of fluids, which could include tea, coffee, sodas and juices is good enough. These notions are false. In order to properly hydrate you need pure, preferably filtered water in quantities that will be effective for your individual body. Most of us lead busy lifestyles, so I would recommend drinking at least 64 ounces (eight x 8 ounce glasses) of water per day, over and above other beverage consumption.

When you should drink? Start when you wake up. Drink a full glass of water before you eat or drink anything else. Hot water will penetrate the cells the fastest. If you want to add a slice of lemon, or the juice of half a lemon, it will provide an immediate infusion of vitamin C and flavor. Remember to stay well hydrated throughout the day. Hydration is an ongoing process. A quick way to tell if you need to increase your water intake is by monitoring the color of your urine. The darker it gets, the more dehydrated you are becoming. Carry a water bottle with you daily. Try and avoid BPA found in plastic water bottles if possible. BPA stands for bisphenol A, an industrial chemical used in the production of some plastics. See a discussion on the negative effects of exposure to BPA under Success Step Nine. BPA exposure should be minimized. Purchase a BPA free water bottle. Glass and stainless steel bottles are a great option too.

Keep in mind that alcohol and caffeine dehydrate the body, and are therefore not adequate replacements for water. Reduce or eliminate these substances, or if you drink them, increase your water intake to combat their effect. Plan to consume about two glasses of water for every glass of coffee or alcohol you drink. Remember, our bodily needs vary based on our exercise level and the weather, so modify your consumption accordingly. Some of the warning signs of dehydration include headaches, muscle cramps, digestive issues, poor concentration, diminished energy, illness, and hunger.

Lesson Three - Keep Moving

Exercise gets your heart pumping, your blood flowing and engages deep breathing, all of which boost your energy. Make space in your day to move your body. The most effective way to ensure that exercise becomes part of your daily and weekly routine is to schedule it as you would a doctor's appointment. Enter it into the family calendar, and then remind everyone that it is an appointment during which you would like not to be disturbed. This has proven to be a very effective tool in my life. I have created a mindset in my family that this is as important to me as their appointments and activities are to them, and should be treated with the same consideration. I realize that this seems like an impossibility to many folks, but a new culture can be developed with persistency.

There are so many ways to incorporate exercise into your day that don't require that hour you think you don't have. I subscribe to the Gaiam wellness channel on cable TV. There are many kinds of classes, from beginner's yoga to advanced cardio routines. I often grab 15-20 minutes to do a simple yoga stretching and breathing class, or start a more advanced cardio class, simply stopping when real life needs me to re-engage. I also purchased a

DVD with twelve minute HIT (High Intensity Training) full body workouts. When that is all the time I have available, I quickly switch it on. Recent studies show that high intensity training elicits tremendous health benefits in the short time it requires to complete, including dramatically reducing hyperglycemia in Type 2 Diabetic patients. The routines include high intensity bursts of exercise ranging from 2-4 minutes, alternating with recovery periods of 60-90 seconds. The routine is then repeated over a 15-20 minute period.

If you have more time, walk alone and enjoy your thoughts, or grab a friend and enjoy some adult time. If you are fighting those few extra pounds we all seem to be carrying, download an app and start to run. Hiring a personal trainer to help you establish several kinds of workouts that you can use throughout your week is well worth the money. In addition to focused exercise, keep moving throughout the day. Try short walks, breathing slowly and deeply. Park in the furthest spot at the market or take the stairs instead of the elevator in a high rise building. All these activities will give you a boost and rejuvenate your energy.

Lesson Four - Avoid Caffeine

Caffeine is a stimulant that will fuel a surge of "energy", followed by a crash that will send you in search of another jolt. When this happens, most people reach for a candy bar or some other form of sugar. This will strap you firmly into that roller coaster seat for a wild ride throughout your day. As documented in a study at Duke University, funded by the National Institutes of Health, appearing in the July/August 2002 issue of Psychosomatic Medicine, caffeine was found to stimulate the excretion of stress hormones. Thinking that you will take a break from your stress with a giant cappuccino and a good book will therefore have the reverse effect. Caffeine consumption has been linked to restlessness, nervousness, and irritability which does little to mitigate the effects of an already stressed system. Additional side effects can include a raise in blood pressure and cholesterol. This does not bode well for people already at risk for heart disease. A great alternative to a caffeinated morning beverage is hot water with lemon, or herbal tea. Green tea and green tea extract (matcha) deliver natural energy without the negative side effects of caffeinated coffee. I use a teaspoon of matcha powder in my morning smoothie.

Lesson Five - Drink Green Smoothies

Try starting your day with a nutrient packed green smoothie (and no, they don't all necessarily look bright green.) I have suggested some recipes in the detox section of the book. Green smoothies, especially those with added protein, give your entire system a wonderful jolt of energy that lasts for hours. Recipes can be customized to address stress, inflammation, detoxification, hydration, balanced daily nutrition and weight loss goals.

Lesson Six - Develop an Energizing Team

Surround yourself with family, friends, co-workers and associates who are positive, energetic "go-getters". The energy is synergistic and dynamic as it flows between like-minded people who embrace daily life with a sense of positivity, adventure and optimism.

Lesson Seven - Find Time for your Passion

My family and friends think I am crazy as I rush from one pursuit to the next, constantly in motion, continuously dreaming up schemes and projects, embracing new challenges and commitments. These pursuits are in the service of the causes I am most passionate about, whether it be children with special needs, animal welfare, mentoring at-risk teens, or wellness coaching. They help stimulate and excite me, while at the same time keeping my energy levels high. You may love drawing, volunteering, gardening, or being a creative force at work. Wherever your passion lies, find time in your day or week to indulge in it. The effects are better than ten cups of coffee!

CHAPTER SUMMARY:

Sleep
Hydrate
Exercise
Avoid Caffeine
Add Green Smoothies
Dynamo Team
Indulge Your Passion

Evaluate Your Inflammation And Imbalance

My mother fought and won her first battle with cancer in 2002. From that point on, both of us became increasingly interested in researching the causes of breast cancer, and what could be done to avoid becoming its victim. One of the most important facts we took away from our ongoing research is the damaging effects of stress on our bodies. A primary reason for this is due to the secretion of stress hormones, most notably cortisol, which creates an inflammatory response in the body. Chronic diseases and illness are linked to inflammation, so it is imperative that we make every attempt in our daily living to reduce stress.

This may seem like an impossibility, given the circumstances of many of our lives. We constantly seem to be in a cortisol induced pattern of fight or flight. I had to consciously reorganize my professional life in order to deal with this challenge, but because I was self-employed I had greater flexibility. For years, I charged out of the house before 8:00 a.m. to drive carpool, and then rushed into work, tearing out again around 4:00 p.m. to collect the kids and get home in time to prepare dinner. Then, back on the road I went to various children's after school activities, meetings with clients, work functions, or simply doing grocery shopping. It was not a sustainable pattern. I have gradually changed my working hours to begin at 10:00 a.m., allowing myself time to exercise, shower, breathe deeply if required, prepare my power house breakfast smoothie, and take my supplements. Delegation of non-essential tasks at home and work has made this possible.

My household responsibilities have become largely that of cooking healthy meals, and meeting the children's individual needs. At work, I have reduced my responsibilities to only the vital essentials, and have largely delegated away the mundane, as well as the things that cause me stress, anxiety or frustration. My husband and I are risk takers when we feel it matters. There is no question that changing my work profile and reducing my availability to employees and clients could have negatively impacted our livelihood. However, in this case it was in the interests of my physical, emotional and spiritual health, and we forged ahead with optimism that it would work out for the best. My husband has become an avid cyclist. He spends a few hours a week in the saddle for many of the same reasons. What good would either of us be to each other, our families or our businesses if we were riddled with stress and unable to function optimally?

We are blessed to live in an age where many companies offer flexible work environments. Many professionals work remotely from home and are able to maintain their employment as long as they meet their required hours. Others are able to job-share. Some couples take turns working day shifts and night shifts so someone is always home as a care-giver. I was able to cut back to three-quarter time. Take the time to evaluate your financial commitments, and then add up the dollars you spend on "wants" but not necessarily needs, and you may find that eliminating non-essential purchases and leisure expenses will actually allow you to reduce working hours without significantly impacting your ability to pay your bills. There are many ways to accomplish the same result. Just be creative.

I have digressed in order to share that tough and scary decisions often need to be made to reduce toxic stress loads that can wreak havoc on your body, as it did on mine. In order to fully appreciate the dangers of *not* addressing stress, the following are *some* of the negative impacts you may experience, including 1) hormonal imbalance; 2) abnormal blood sugar swings, which can lead to pre-diabetes or diabetes; 3) weight gain, full-blown obesity, and metabolic syndrome; 4) anxiety, depression, impaired memory; 5) sleep issues; 6) heart disease; 7) gastrointestinal issues. My inability to easily lose weight is directly related to hormonal imbalance, primarily from my cortisol levels, driven by my stress. If you have concerns about your cortisol levels, there are home kits for self-testing. A simple saliva sample, collected at various times during the day and night and mailed to a lab will give you the answers you need to determine whether you are within the normal range or spiraling out of control. This test has been one of my most valuable resources regarding managing my cortisol levels in my daily struggle to keep my own stress minimized.

Engaging in activities that address the mind-body connection can also powerfully reduce the symptoms of stress and inflammation. These may include yoga, meditation, tai chi, qigong, breathing exercises, and even journaling your thoughts, feelings and aspirations. All of these practices engage in a process of focusing on the points of stress in your body, and then consciously attempting to reduce, and preferably eliminate them. If time and resources are a challenge, all of the above can be attempted at home with videos, or through following a class or demonstration online or on cable T.V. I have been doing this successfully for years.

THE STRESS BUSTERS CHALLENGE:

Start with one day a week. See if you can consciously stop in your tracks at the moment of heightened stress. Complete an entry on this page, and adopt one strategy to alleviate the stress.

I FEEL STRESSED	REMEDY				RESULT
Day & Time	Yoga	Meditation	Breathing	Journal Entry	Result

SUPERCHARGED MOM

What's Your Gut Feeling?

I had stomach ache for years, literally. I went through the obligatory colonoscopy and endoscopy process recommended by the gastroenterologist. All that the doctor could uncover (luckily) was the fact that I had inflamed my insides with over-the-counter painkillers. This was certainly an important piece of information - a catalyst for me to stop relying on painkillers as a band aid, to try and discover the root cause of the problem. It was suggested that I suffered from Irritable Bowel Syndrome (IBS), and I went home armed with a prescription for reflux which was supposed to mitigate the discomfort, but in fact did absolutely nothing at all. At this point I decided to rely on natural remedies. As my journey to health began, and my foods became cleaner, I really believed I would experience an easing of the discomfort. I did not. I then decided to remove gluten from my diet. I definitely felt a difference. The stomach aches, bloating and gas all but disappeared, although I still experienced discomfort under my left ribcage, and was suffering from tremendous fatigue, making it almost impossible to get through the day. In desperation I consulted with a functional medicine doctor. After a battery of tests, he discovered that I had an intestinal parasite. Three days into taking an antibiotic the relief was palpable. I turned to my husband and said "I feel like I have my life back!" An additional test revealed mild leaky gut (another term for Increased Intestinal Permeability), necessitating a regimen of supplements for healing. The reason for divulging all of this is to give you some insight into the fact that there is often no single cure or approach to healing certain conditions. It requires a multi-faceted approach, harnessing the powerful combination of several disciplines, including mainstream medicine, functional or integrative medicine, and natural approaches to healing. (For an explanation of functional and integrative medicine, visit the resource section.)

It is no coincidence that I received the additional leaky gut diagnosis. As a stressed out parent of non-typical children, I am sometimes amazed that I do not have many more ailments in my medical files. Remember the conversation about the destructive nature of stress? Clinical studies have proven the link between chronic psychological stress and intestinal permeability. The effects of this condition can severely impact our health, as the explanation further on in this chapter details.

Running the gamut from IBS to reflux to a parasite to leaky gut was a very frustrating experience. You are probably just as frustrated by all of these terms. Below you will find a synopsis of some of the most common culprits to intestinal discomfort. If you suspect that you could be suffering from one or more of these, I recommend working with an holistic practitioner or functional or integrative medical doctor who can prescribe the necessary testing, as well as the supplement regimen (or dietary restrictions) to combat the effects. In some instances the affliction can be healed - in some cases, life-long dietary and life-style adjustments are necessary. (There are many chiropractors, homeopaths, and naturopaths who can provide testing kits too.)

Gut Feelings

Irritable Bowel Syndrome (IBS): Irritable bowel syndrome can cause abdominal pain, bloating, gas, cramps, diarrhea and/or constipation. It does not damage the intestinal tract like an inflammatory bowel disease, but can still negatively impact daily life. Doctors usually prescribe medications to control it, but in my case, diet and lifestyle changes eliminated it.

Gluten Sensitivity: I highly recommend eliminating gluten from your diet if possible. Gluten can be highly inflammatory. In addition, you could be experiencing a reaction to it without realizing it. In my case, my years long battle with sinus congestion and post nasal drip vanished the minute I eliminated gluten, as did the bloating and gas after meals that included gluten. A genetic test, ordered by my functional medicine doctor, clearly showed that my body responded negatively to gluten.

Increased Intestinal Permeability, also known as Leaky Gut Syndrome: The gastrointestinal tract has a single layer of cells separating it from the surrounding organs and abdominal cavity. The intestinal tract is in the critical business of separating nutrients from toxins, and then sending toxic waste into the colon for elimination. It is very important that these toxins, and other matter, be contained and not be allowed to escape into the abdominal cavity. When this layer of cells widens, it creates gaps that allow the intestinal wall to be breached. The contents of the gastrointestinal tract can then seep into the body, bypassing the routine process of absorption through cell transfer (of only the desirable elements). This leak triggers an inflammatory response, resulting in a host of diseases, including the two described below.

The following two conditions are worth mentioning because of the vast numbers of people affected by them. If you suspect that you or a family member could be suffering from either, you should consult a medical doctor at your earliest opportunity. Both of these conditions require life-long management and care:

Crohn's and Ulcerative Colitis: These are inflammatory bowel diseases, triggered by the body's immune system. The exact reason for onset is not yet fully understood. Some of the symptoms include diarrhea, rectal bleeding, abdominal pain, cramps, fatigue, reduced appetite, and weight loss.

Celiac Disease: An autoimmune disorder that is triggered by the consumption of gluten, and results in the immune system attacking the small intestine, damaging the villi and making it harder to absorb much needed nutrients into the body. Some of the telltale signs, as listed by the Celiac Disease Foundation on their website at www.celiac.org include, but are not limited to: fatigue, bone or joint pain, depression or anxiety, tingling numbness in the hands and feet, canker sores inside the mouth, an itchy skin rash.

The saying "You Are What You Eat" really rings true. The foods we consume not only give us life, they also determine our health by becoming either essential building blocks or harmful toxins when ingested. The stomach and intestinal tract is where the absorption takes place. If the health of these organs is compromised, it can affect the body's ability to absorb the nutrients it needs not only to survive and function but to thrive and be healthy.

SUPERCHARGED MOM

Take Your Emotional Temperature

Poor emotional conditioning leads to exhaustion, stress, depression, impaired communication, and marital problems. Our responsibility as parents is to admit when our emotions are manifesting as one or more of the above symptoms, and then to seek help. I spent a long time in denial of my emotional pain, and it was leading to a dark and dangerous place. When parenting special needs and learning impaired children, the emotional pain comes and goes in waves. There are times when the children are stable and flourishing, and our pain is temporarily suppressed. Then there comes a time when the children are facing hurdles once again, and we hurt right along with them. I actually think we hurt more than they do by presuming they are experiencing things to which they may, in fact, be oblivious. I will share an example. In an interview with a mother, she shared how painful it was to see the neighborhood girls playing on the court outside her home, while her special needs daughter of the same age remained on the fringe, unable to participate. I know her daughter - she is a bubbly and dear child. Do I think that she is experiencing pain by not being included in this social circle? I do not. Does that lessen the pain her mother feels? It does not.

When my Aspie boy was bullied in middle school by his non-disabled peers, and we decided to remove him from the school to protect him physically and emotionally, it was such a painful experience. He did not understand why he was being pulled out of the school his siblings were attending. He was the victim, yet he felt he was being punished. He became very depressed, and it manifested in a physical reaction that necessitated a brief hospital stay and several months of medical intervention. My other children were experiencing terrible pain at seeing their beloved sibling being mistreated and misunderstood, and their tears carved a gulley into our hearts that has hardened into eternal scars. To this day I cannot recount that period in our lives without choking up.

How did I overcome times of incredible emotional pain? Faith, resilience, and the love and support of our team. Throughout the periods in our family's journey when the pain escalated, we tried really hard to put our faith in our Creator, that He had a plan for our children and our family that we may not have been seeing or understanding in that moment, but that would ultimately be revealed. Then, eventually a new path opened up, and we looked back and realized that the previous incident or challenge was the dress rehearsal for something much better, that was just over the horizon. In my son's case a new school placement in the middle of sixth grade seemed a recipe for disaster, but in fact was a blessing. In his new school, a safe and nurturing environment with case workers who carefully monitored his emotional, social and educational well-being, he flourished beyond anything we could have imagined.

That being said, it seems we are never quite done in the pain department. Some of it is integrally related to shame and embarrassment, and some to circumstantial behaviors and situations. There are challenges that seem to run across multiple diagnoses, like delayed maturity, abnormal speech patterns, socially inappropriate behaviors, potty training that seems to go on forever, to name just a few. These are some of the *invisible* features of children whose outward appearance may appear indistinguishable from their non-disabled peers. However, to a parent, these issues can cause excessive emotional stress as the battle wages to catch the children up to age-appropriate levels before they do themselves irreparable harm socially. My special needs children have all, at one time or another, had an innate ability to embarrass themselves, often just when things seem to be running smoothly. It may be calling out someone publically for being mean, or ranting in an online forum. It could be throwing down a baseball bat in the middle of a game and walking off the field. No matter the circumstance, and irrespective of how empathetic and understanding the audience, our instinctive response as parents is shame and pain. And it cuts really deeply.

Once again, let me stress how vital it is that your partner be your strongest team member during these periods of your life. If your marriage is in jeopardy, your first priority is to address that with professional help. This could be in the form of a licensed therapist or a clergy member who is also a trained relationship counselor, and many are. Over the years I have often heard the statistic that over 80% of marriages in which there is a child with special needs end in divorce. This may also have crossed your mind. However, I have not yet found any compelling data to suggests that this is accurate. In addition, I have not found any conclusive evidence that parents of special needs children who divorce do so as a *result* of their child's diagnosis. There is a natural inclination to infer that parents of special needs children divorce because of the challenges of parenting these kids, when in fact, it may be *despite* them!

In light of the above I came across the results of a study directed by Dr. Brian Freedman, Ph.D. clinical director of the Center for Autism and Related Disorders at the Kennedy Krieger Institute in Baltimore. This study clearly refutes that the 80% theory universally affects special needs families. "… his research team found that 64 percent of children with an autism spectrum disorder (ASD) belong to a family with two married biological or adoptive parents, compared with 65 percent of children who do not have an ASD." In addition, "Previous research speaks to the fact that parenting a child with autism is stressful, and it puts pressure on the marriage. Dr. Freedman noted that past studies have found couples with a child with autism experience more stress in their marriage than couples with typically developing children or couples with children with other types of developmental disabilities, such as Down syndrome. Mothers of children with autism report more depression than those with typically developing children, while fathers report they deal with the stress by distancing themselves and becoming less involved with the family.[2]" I found it remarkable and reaffirming that despite admissions of incredible stress and depression, there is only a one percent difference in the marriage statistics of parents with children on the spectrum, versus families facing other diagnoses. It is also encouraging to note that 65% of the couples in this study were still married, as opposed to only 20% if the 80% theory holds true.

The bottom line is that, no matter the circumstances, if you are in pain and feel unable to manage the consequences on your own, or as a couple, do not delay seeking help. Your emotional health and stability is of critical importance. You are the anchor that keeps your family from spinning out of control, and they all depend on you. You cannot take care of them if you are not taking care of yourself first.

---

[2] (https://www.kennedykrieger.org/overview/news/80-percent-autism-divorce-rate-debunked-first-its-kind-scientific-study

SUPERCHARGED MOM

Part Three — The How:

PATHWAYS TO SUCCESS

De-Junking The Pantry

Living with a child on the spectrum dictates that life needs to unfold with a sense of order, with the certainty that everything will be the same, or as expected, day in and day out. Routines are scripted, and these children are primed ahead for events that vary from this daily routine, such as vacations or the need for a sudden appointment. My household was no exception. There came the time, however, where I intentionally deviated, knowing full well that chaos would ensue. I had decided it was time to clean out the pantry in order to clean up my entire family's diets. It was impossible for me to improve the quality of my health through nutrition if my household was not stocked and equipped for such a lifestyle change. It is not feasible to cook and shop separately for one family member when running a household of children with competing needs.

I hired a fellow IIN® graduate to help me, and we set to work cleaning out the pantry, fridge and freezer. Out went breakfast cereals, which are loaded with added sugar, artificial food colors, and are often made from an extruded paste with little to no nutritional value. Next went cookies, white breads and bagels, processed sauces, lunch meats and sausages filled with nitrates, boxes of macaroni and cheese, chicken nuggets, various frozen foods, margarine and non-organic dairy products. Armed with a new grocery list, I headed off to the nearest Whole Foods Market to purchase a new pantry of "clean" foods.

The term "clean" foods refers to foods that are unprocessed, consisting of real, whole foods, with minimal added ingredients. If you want to maintain a clean diet, your pantry and fridge will likely contain the following:

1. Fresh fruits and vegetables, organic whenever possible. If you need to make choices, consult the dirty dozen list in the resource section of the book to help you identify which fruits and vegetables have the highest toxic load.
2. Healthy fats and oils such as olive, coconut, avocado, sesame and nut oils
3. Whole grains such as oats, brown rice, quinoa, bulgur, millet
4. Whole wheat and/or gluten free pasta
5. Home-made or organic breads
6. Breakfast oatmeal and unsweetened granola
7. Organic, free-range eggs
8. Home-made pasta sauce
9. Nut, rice and/or coconut milks
10. Organic dairy products
11. Organic, grass-fed meat and poultry

12. Wild caught, low mercury fish (see list in the resource section)

13. Beans, nuts and legumes (I use canned chick peas and beans from Eden as their brand uses BPA free cans)

14. Home-made salsa, guacamole and dips (hummus is my favorite)

15. Clean condiments such as mustards, healthy mayonnaise, home-made barbecue sauce, pickles, sauerkraut, pickled vegetables (so easy to make), applesauce

16. Organic tortilla and corn chips are preferable to potato chips and other processed snacks

17. Clean snack bars with limited ingredients, and unsweetened dried fruits especially raisins, apricots, and dates which can be used as natural sweeteners for baking and cooking

18. Nut butters with no added sugars

19. Protein powders for healthy smoothies and shakes

School lunch boxes obviously become more of a problem when trying to maintain a clean eating household. Fortunately there are many practical yet innovative ideas to be found on the internet. I had to switch my children over to bento box style lunches. They were used to a lunch that included a sandwich, several processed snacks, and fruit juices. Now they had to be satisfied with sandwiches, or tubs of chicken strips and vegetable crudités, hummus with tortilla chips, smoothies, tubs of sliced or whole fresh fruit, and a water bottle. (See some recommendations in the resource section.)

It wasn't pretty to begin with. Going cold-turkey was rough. My children and husband left home one day, and arrived back a few hours later to find a very different way of eating had been instituted, with no prior warning. For months they resisted the change - they fought and screamed, but then something incredible unfolded. My husband and two of the children suffered from asthma. Both children frequently used the nebulizer for seasonal allergies. The other two children suffered from eczema. My youngest son had caught molluscum contagiosum that I had tried unsuccessfully to get rid of. He also had yearly bouts of strep throat. Suddenly, we began to notice that no-one had complained of any ailments for a while. No headaches, stomach aches, the molluscum disappeared with the help of a multi-vitamin, probiotic and fish oil regimen. My youngest got through the winter months with no strep, and the asthma and eczema symptoms disappeared. He also declared that he no longer needed his ADD meds at school as he was doing much better, thank you very much! My husband and I have found that we have much larger reserves of energy. We have both lost some needed pounds without dieting. None of my children are over-weight. I rarely experience headaches, and my stuffy nose is a thing of the past.

As I cooked, and subtly discussed the benefits of all the new foods with my family, everyone began to connect the dots. They would arrive home from play dates and birthday parties complaining that they felt ill from the effects of the soda, cakes and processed foods they had consumed. Along with me, they started to experience the before and after effects of a clean diet, and now they too sought the benefits. It has not always been plain sailing. There are still days where no-one is willing to try a new dish, or I field complaints that there is "nothing to eat in this house", when in fact the fridge is filled with home-cooked food. However, if I can maintain an environment in which we are all eating clean 80-90% of the time, the minimal amount of other foods we consume is not enough to mitigate the benefits.

Even though the focus of this book is on the health of us parents, some important research is briefly worth mentioning that has made the link between nutrition, food additives, food toxicity, and the explosion of various disabilities and conditions, including Autism, ADD/ADHD, asthma, skin conditions such as eczema and psoriasis, in addition to documented links between food triggers and allergies. Since World War II there has literally been epidemic-like surges in these diagnoses. The question of *why* has been the subject of years of research by scientists, chemists, doctors and professionals in many disciplines. Alarming links have been made, some going back decades, to the fact that as Western nations have become more industrialized, our food chains have become more toxic. The introduction of massive, factory-scale farming and rearing of animals for consumption has led to farming practices that are not only offensive to our moral and humane sensibilities, but have necessitated the use of massive amounts of chemicals and antibiotics. Those tainted ingredients then get sent to factories, where additional synthetic chemicals are added, and what emerges are brightly colored, attractively packaged "Franken-Foods" beckoning to unsuspecting consumers from the supermarket shelves, fridges and freezers. From the Baby Boomer generation onwards, we have been the guinea pigs in what is turning out to be a devastating experiment. In their singular quest for profit, large corporations have stripped away our rights to even gain insight and understanding into the contents of our foods. And, if this is not destructive enough, they have loaded our household cleaners and personal care products with even more damaging substances (more on this later in the next section on detoxing). It is interesting to note how corporations are suddenly taking more interest in the contents of their products as consumers demand more organic choices, and cleaner foods and household products. As they see the burgeoning demand, the billions of dollars to be made, accommodating the marketplace is finally pushing these large corporations for more transparency in their quest for more market share. The response is still infinitesimal, but hopefully the free market place will lead to a future of clean, safe foods, personal care items and household cleaners of the quality our grandmothers may have used.

As parents, we are automatic advocates for our family's well-being, and as you will learn in this section and the next, eliminating some of the most prevalent toxins from the entire family's diet can powerfully impact and benefit everyone's health, as it did in our home. When I de-junked my own pantry, the foods containing the following went out first.

Artificial colors: The following excerpt from the results of a clinical study says it all! "The consumption of synthetic food colors, and their ability to bind with body proteins, can have significant immunological consequences. This consumption can activate the inflammatory cascade, can result in the induction of intestinal permeability to large antigenic molecules, and could then lead to cross-reactivities, autoimmunities, and even neurobehavioral disorders. The Centers for Disease Control (CDC) recently found a 41% increase in diagnoses of ADHD in boys of high-school age during the past decade. More shocking is the legal amount of artificial colorants allowed by the FDA in the foods, drugs, and cosmetics that we consume and use every day. The consuming public is largely unaware of the perilous truth behind the deceptive allure of artificial color." (Altern Ther Health Med. 2015;21 Suppl 1:52-62. Immune reactivity to food coloring. Vojdani A, Vojdani C. PMID: 25599186.)

In a summary by the Center for Science in the Public Interest (CSPI), additional side effects are listed as kidney tumors (Blue 1 in animal studies), thyroid tumors (Red 3), allergic responses and hyperactivity (Yellow 5), adrenal gland, kidney and testicular tumors (Yellow 6). (https://cspinet.org/resource/summary-studies-food-dyes)

Added sugars: Sugar (sucrose) has close to 60 different names, and appears in our food and beverages under those guises, sometimes multiple times in the ingredient listing for just one food! When you add up the grams of the various sugars mentioned, the combined quantity can trump all the other ingredients in that food stuff. Learning how to recognize the various names of sugar will enable you to control the quantities consumed by your family. Some of these names include dextrose, glucose, maltose, mannitol, sorbitol, barley malt, molasses and many more! In order to avoid falling prey to such tactics implemented by the food industry on a non-suspecting population of consumers, try and eat clean by avoiding all processed foods, fruit juices and sodas.

MSG and Aspartame: Both are excitotoxins. In a study published by the National Institute of Health, the ingestion of MSG was shown to increase levels of free radicals, and accelerate the onset of oxidative stress. What does this mean? Atoms are bound together by electrons to create stability in our cell molecules.

When these bonds are weakened they split, resulting in free radicals. If left unchecked by antioxidants, they can destroy healthy surrounding cells creating damage in our bodies. Oxidative stress is the result. In addition, MSG has been demonstrated in studies to have a toxic effect on the neurons in our brains, which can result in swelling and injury. (Int J Clin Exp Med. 2009; 2(4): 329-336, Nov 2009. Jennifer S. Xiong, Debbie Branign and Minghau Li).

Nitrates and Nitrites: These are preservatives found in processed foods, most notably lunch meats and hot dogs. In an article dated June 23, 2015 the Environmental Working Group cautioned that "Manufacturers add nitrates and nitrites to foods such as cured sandwich meats, bacon, salami or sausages to give them color and to prolong their shelf life. When added to processed foods in this way, both nitrates and nitrites can form nitrosamines in the body, which can increase your risk of developing cancer."

BVO (Brominated Vegetable Oil): This product is used in sodas and sports drinks to bind the ingredients together and prevent them from separating, as oil and water do, when combined. When consumed in large doses it can prove toxic. It is also used as a flame retardant! BVO is banned for consumption in Europe and Japan. In 2014 both Coca Cola and Pepsico agreed to begin phasing out their use of BVO in fruit flavored and sports drinks. To date this has not in fact happened with all products containing BVO.

BPA (Bisphenol A): BPA is a chemical used to harden plastics. It leaches into the substances it contains, and when heated does so in higher doses. Animal studies show exposure increases the risk of obesity, type 2 diabetes, a variety of cancers, hyperactivity, and cardiovascular disease.

Phthalates: These chemicals are used to create flexibility in plastics. Leaching causes endocrine disruption, affects male reproductive development, and can subject people to increase risks of asthma and eczema.

I don't want to scare you into starving yourself or your family by telling you that there are several more toxic substances that you should be aware of when you make your supermarket rounds. If you are interested in researching them, a wealth of material can be found on the internet, along with scientific studies located at www.pubmed.gov.

There is no down side to moving your household to a clean eating model. It can successfully be phased in little by little, or in faster stages. Ultimately, everyone wins. There are no losers when you seek to improve the quality of your own health - and take your family along on the journey.

SUCCESS STEP TEN:

Detoxing Your Body And Life

You have gotten some help at home, are regimenting your sleeping habits, squeezing in some exercise, and you've cleaned out the pantry. You are still feeling lousy. What do you do? You are ready to detox things from your body and soul that steal your energy and vitality. This process involves not only the physical purging of toxins and allergens, but includes an evaluation of situations and relationships that may be adding large doses of conscious and unconscious stress to your already overloaded immune system. I intuitively always knew that stress was a driver of chronic illness because I felt it manifesting in my body in a variety of ways. I did not fully appreciate the extent of the damage that it could unleash until my functional medicine doctor ordered a battery of tests. I had passed the detox stage, had already eliminated so much from my diet, was exercising five days a week, sleeping well, and had my daily schedule somewhat under control. However, when those test results came back and I saw my elevated levels of inflammation, I realized that even I had a long road ahead. Additionally, I discovered that I was suffering from heavy metal poisoning, specifically mercury and aluminum. It is not enough to address all these factors and assume perfect or even adequate health. The long-term effects of maintaining toxic levels of food, stress, chemicals and negative emotions trapped in our bodies does not necessarily respond to healing instantaneously. It also may persist *despite* our best efforts to eradicate it, and may require the expertise of a trained health care professional, especially a functional or integrative medical doctor.

The focus on toxicity in the body has only in recent decades become a mainstream concept in our Western society, spearheaded by functional and integrative medicine, as well as holistic practitioners. However, in the traditional medicines of the ancient Eastern cultures, the body's ability to detoxify itself physically, intellectually and emotionally is of primary importance. If one is out of balance, Eastern medicine believes that this lack of harmony between the body's systems is the root cause of a host of ailments. In Traditional Chinese Medicine balancing one's energy, the Qi, is essential for good health. In Ayurvedic medicine of ancient India, the main objective is the clearing out from the body of all undigested foods, and toxins in the lymphatic system – toxic waste.

The benefits of detoxing or cleansing your body include strengthening your immune system, boosting your energy, improving your moods, reducing anxiety and depression, sharpening your focus, reducing and often eliminating food cravings, weight loss, better digestion, and a reduction in physical pain and inflammation. With that list in mind, what do you have to lose? Let's discuss a progression of steps you can take to start feeling lighter physically and emotionally.

Detox your Body

A detox or elimination diet can help you figure out what foods may be obstacles to your progress. There are several versions, and you can select one that you feel you can undertake with minimal added stress. The most basic is a combination of juicing or blending, along with a simple diet of greens, low carbohydrate vegetables, healthy fats and proteins. The next step is to slowly add back a list of foods, one at a time. Since we have in theory eliminated the foods that most commonly trigger allergenic or negative responses in our bodies, we can figure out what the root cause of some of our symptoms may be if any of those symptoms return when we add a particular food back into our diet. Each step needs to be evaluated, and if you start to feel tired, or stuffy nosed, or bloated and gassy, or experience any other undesirable effect on your body, you may have found one of your trigger foods. This process is called an elimination diet.

The most complex detoxing process involves juice fasting, and I would not recommend undertaking this unless you have the time, and some help at home. The side effects can be more severe, and you may feel unwell for an extended period of time. Working with a health coach or integrative medical practitioner can be very helpful through this process. My most trusted detox diets are those designed by medical doctors, and I would most certainly advise you to pick one system and follow it. I have used this process extensively to assist me with my healing. The following are some of the basic concepts to understand and some of the steps you can take when undertaking a detox or elimination diet:

Step One

Your kidneys are going to play an important role in the detoxification process. To assist them, it is important to stay well hydrated. Maintaining your body in an alkaline pH state as much as possible will also help. Disease thrives in an acidic body. Focus on consuming alkaline foods such as leafy green vegetables, gluten free whole grains (rice, quinoa, buckwheat, millet, amaranth and teff), beans, fruit, drinking plenty of water or green/herbal teas, and use lemon or apple cider vinegar as condiments. Avoid acidic foods like meat and poultry, dairy products, refined and processed foods, sugar, alcohol and drugs, coffee and sodas. (See the resource section for a more comprehensive list.) You can also purchase a pH strip from a drug store. Testing your saliva with it in the early morning and late afternoon will help you access your levels.

Step Two

Enjoy a glass of hot water with lemon on awaking in the morning. This combination hydrates, is alkalizing, and begins the detoxification process by flushing out toxins. It also assists with healthy digestion.

Step Three

Introduce a green smoothie as your breakfast. You will need a high speed blender to adequately break down these ingredients. A basic green smoothie blend is as follows (see additional recipes in the resource section):

BASIC GREEN ENERGY DRINK

1 Cup of Water
½ Cup Unsweetened Almond, Rice, Hemp or Coconut
Milk
2 Cups Organic Kale, Spinach or Mixed Greens
Juice of 1 Lemon (Optional)
1 Organic Green Apple with Skin and Pits Included
½ Frozen Banana
2 Organic Dates Pitted (Optional for Added Sweetness)
1" Piece of Fresh Ginger Root
A Scoop of Protein Powder (Optional)

Step Four

Choose clean and simple snacks for between meals if needed such as vegetables with guacamole or hummus dips, or a small handful of nuts (no more than a dozen, or half an ounce).

Step Five

For lunch and dinner select a large green salad with two cups of greens, a cup of raw (or a half cup of cooked) low carbohydrate vegetables, a healthy fat such as an olive oil and vinegar dressing, a quarter avocado (or 3 tablespoons of nuts or seeds) and a small serving of a clean protein such as 5 ounces organic, free range poultry, or wild caught low-mercury fish (sardines, salmon, butterfish, flounder, scallops, shrimp, tilapia, trout, Pacific sole, to name just a few of the most popular). Use pure spices, as opposed to blends (that may contain sugar, hidden chemicals and gluten) and fresh herbs to season your food and dressings. I would remain off eggs, beans, legumes, tofu, and tempeh for the first five days too (my reasons follow).

Step Six

After five days, begin adding back foods one at a time for a three day period each to access your body's reaction. Many people are sensitive to eggs, for example, and just don't realize it until they start adding it back through an elimination diet. I always thought I had an allergenic response to the sulfites in red wine. Whenever I dined out and enjoyed a glass, I would wake up with congestion. However, when I eliminated gluten from my diet the congestion disappeared. Thereafter I tried a glass of red wine and experienced no negative side effects. If you have been a notorious junk food eater, and sugar has been your vice, you may want to add high sugar foods last. At that point, you may find that you no longer have the same craving for them as you did before you started detoxing. You may also experience specific responses in your body when reintroducing sugar. When I consume sugar over and above the natural sugars in my morning smoothie from fruit, my head instantly starts to spin. By the way, that does not always deter me from eating chocolate! I wish that it would.

Our bodies can become toxic from other sources too. Most people don't realize that the skin is our body's largest organ. Conventional cosmetics are loaded with harmful substances that increase with long-term exposure. If you think of all the products we use, from soaps and shampoos, to moisturizers, deodorants and sunscreens, our bodies have been absorbing a host of strange and sometimes toxic substances since infancy. In my efforts to reduce toxicity in my body and my family's, I switched to a line of personal care items that *do not* contain 99% of the ingredients listed below:

THE DETOX CHECK-LIST

Parabens, preservatives used in personal care items: Animal studies have discovered it to be an endocrine disruptor.

Phthalates, used to bind ingredients in personal care products: Animal studies have discovered it to be an endocrine disruptor.

Triclosan, an anti-bacterial agent found in personal care products such as soaps and toothpaste: Banned by the FDA in September 2016 for being ineffective, and promoting antibiotic resistant bacteria to grow and flourish.

Resorcinol, most commonly found in hair dyes and dermatological treatments: Most common symptoms of overexposure are the irritation of eyes, skin, nose, throat, and upper respiratory system.

Hydroquinone, a skin whitening agent: Banned by the FDA in 2006 as a potential carcinogen.

MIT (Methylisothiazolinone), a preservative used in personal care products: It is a cytotoxin, and can also elicit widespread dermatological allergic responses.

Mineral Oil is used as a laxative, and in dermatological products: Exposure to low grade, industrial and impure oils, has been linked to skin cancer. The concern is that the use of impure or low grade oils can toxify these products.

Oxybenzone, used in sunscreens: Is linked in studies to hormone disruption, and has been found to elicit allergenic dermatological responses.

Artificial Dyes and Synthetic Colors: Several colors are still approved for use in personal care products, as well as food and beverages.

Heavy Metals, like Mercury and Lead: Found in some make-up products, accumulation in the body creates toxicity over time. This can affect the functioning of major bodily systems including the brain, the nervous system, the respiratory system, and the reproductive system.

An excellent place to find out more about these toxins and which products contain them is on the Environmental Working Group's website at www.ewg.org. I use their databases to check up on everything from a non-toxic window cleaner to a safe sunscreen.

Detox Your Life

You cannot have an overwhelming number of commitments and do justice to your own health and that of your family. Learn to say NO. Select only activities and commitments that are affirming, uplifting and energizing, and help propel your life forward. Seek opportunities to help others who may be on the same journey. When you give, you receive, sometimes ten-fold. More importantly, put your disabled or affected children front and center unapologetically. Don't be afraid to be selective in determining what to participate in and what to steer clear of. Stress is toxic, and one of the core principals in maintaining your health is to keep stress to a minimum.

I will give you an example from my life. We had booked flights to attend a family event in Florida. We already knew that our Aspie guy did not embrace traveling. However, this was an important event in celebration of my niece, and we had been priming him that we were all going. A few days before the flight he started with the "I am not getting on that plane" routine. We tried everything in our arsenal to work through the block to no avail. Eventually my husband pulled the trigger and cancelled our two flights. He would go alone with the other three children. My heart was heavy. I really wanted to be with the family coming in from far and near. I had bought the dress and was ready to celebrate. It was just as well that I stayed. During that weekend, as a result of staying home, I discovered my son doing something that could have been damaging and destructive had I not caught it.

Asperger's children do not have very good filters, and often head innocently into unchartered waters out of sheer curiosity.

This was one such instance. It reaffirmed to my husband and I that, as vigilant as you may be in trying to shield special needs children from accessing dangerous places on the Internet, perpetuating damaging behaviors, forging unhealthy friendships, and all manner of other things, it still may not be enough! Let's take friendships as an example. Children with a variety of diagnoses are poor judges of character. In addition, they may be more easily hurt by their peers, or negatively influenced by them. We have always tried to understand the friendship dynamics of our affected children, and have often found it necessary to delineate heathy relationships from destructive and hurtful ones – a skill that they are not adept at.

What began as a seemingly unnecessary and frustrating sacrifice as a result of my son's needs turned out to be a unique and important window into something going on in his life that was important we became aware of. There have been many more instances where we have had to decline participating in activities or events, often of close friends and family. It requires embracing a mindset that we are doing this out of love for ourselves and our children. Perhaps I take away from that the lesson that in avoiding a predictably stressful situation, we gleaned other benefits in addition to simply avoiding stress. I took solace in this, despite missing a family function, because I have learned that the consequences of being dragged into stressful circumstances against our better judgment are extremely toxic.

Detox Your Relationships

If you have toxic relationships that drive your stress levels up, put those relationships on hold, or eliminate them all together. We moved our family across a continent in order to eliminate interference in the decisions we were making regarding our children. Most families do not have that option. You do have a choice, though, in who you allow to affect your life, and in what capacity. It is certainly worth commending and celebrating our children's milestones. However, in families with special needs children, those accomplishments may look entirely different from families with typically developing children. You may find yourself faced with a friend or associate who takes great pleasure in continuously boasting about their child's sporting or academic prowess, while for you, an uneventful day without any meltdowns is a major achievement. You may find the comparisons humiliating, embarrassing, depressing or stressful. In that instance your relationship with that person may be toxifying your life, and you may need to distance yourself simply for self-preservation. Once again, your mindset may need to adjust in order to embrace this decision as one of self-love – a vital component in effective healing.

Detox Your Environment

Environmental toxins are responsible for creating many health hazards. In our home, asthma and eczema were exacerbated by environmental factors. During my cleaning out phase, I switched all my household cleaners and detergents to natural, non-toxic brands. That, coupled with dietary changes, led to the eradication or dramatic improvement of those conditions.

If your family suffers from respiratory ailments and seasonal allergies, clean air is essential in your home. There are several domestic air filtration systems available. They all use different mechanisms, and outcomes and prices vary. Find a system that seems appropriate in combatting your health concerns.

Water filtration systems are also a worthwhile investment. As we continue to see instances and effects, across the country, of polluted drinking water, we should be cognizant of the quality of the drinking water in our own homes. In addition to toxic pollutants that can affect local water supplies, drinking water in general contains fluctuating levels of chlorine, fluoride, and other added chemicals. A water filtration system attached to an incoming water source in a kitchen, such as a reverse osmosis system, is a simple and inexpensive solution. These are freely available at your neighborhood home supply store. A whole house filtration system will regulate bath and shower water quality too, but requires a more serious capital outlay.

The Detox Challenge:

Each month replace one household item with a cleaner, less toxic substitute:

OUT WITH...	IN WITH...
Example: Shampoo containing sulfates	OGX Shampoo (available at most stores including Walmart)

SUPERCHARGED MOM

Get Cooking

Preparing meals from scratch gives you control over your health and the health of everyone in your household. That being said, it is one of the first sacrifices we make as mothers of special needs children, because our time is already stretched. However, there are some basic tools in my toolbox that I employ to make this happen in my home, and they are as follows.

1. Communicate with your children: Ask them what they would like for dinners. Buy-in can make life so much easier. Integrate their kid-friendly suggestions into your meals, while upping the ante when it comes to using clean and healthy ingredients. I do not suggest that pasta and cheese pizza feature on the nightly menu, but agreeing to pizza if they in turn agree to add an extra vegetable of their choice to the topping, may be a step in the right direction.

It is important that the meals include healthy dishes the entire family are willing to participate in. It is of equal importance that everyone learns that meals can be an adventure, and that when we are on an adventure, we open ourselves up to experiencing new things. I will now unapologetically admit that the way I handled this was to start out completely subversively. I purchased cookbooks that involved steaming and pureeing a variety of vegetables, and then hiding them in the food. I stored the purees in the freezer in glass ramekins in 1-2 cup portions. As I cooked, I added these to different recipes. After my family complimented a meal that included a previously vetoed vegetable, I would break the news to them that they had just consumed copious amounts of cauliflower, and "wasn't that great?"! Of course, as you can imagine, the first response was always "EEEEUUUUW!" However, they had painted themselves into a corner by admitting freely that they had enjoyed the meal, so I would add it to the healthy meal rotation and they would eat it again. This tactic helped elevate my own health tremendously. It ensured that on most nights I could prepare one meal, rather than being a short order line cook and making a different item for each child. That relieved stress and saved time. It also meant that all of us were consuming meals of higher nutritional value and lower caloric count. Now, I don't specifically advocate a lifestyle dependent on monitoring caloric intake, but if you are going to feel satiated after a meal laden with clean proteins, healthy fats, and tons of vegetable sides, it is certainly a win-win situation. This leads to the next point.

2. Go for nutrient density, not just caloric content: There is a vast difference between a 100 calorie snack pack of pretzels or cookies, and 100 calories of fruit and vegetables.   The difference lies in how your body responds to these foods and what it decides to do with them during the digestive process.   When we consume fresh fruits and vegetables, nuts, seeds, legumes, healthy fats and pure proteins, our body absorbs the necessary building blocks like amino acids, minerals, and vitamins that it needs for all of our systems to function properly.   When we introduce a synthetic product, created in a laboratory from chemicals, such as Thiamine Mononitrate (a synthetic B1 vitamin found in SnackWells 100 calorie snacks), we are essentially ingesting a foreign substance.   It is not water soluble and therefore does not pass through our systems.   Instead, it accumulates in our kidneys, liver and fat tissues.   A build-up in the liver can be toxic and lead to severe damage over time.   In addition, because of its synthetic nature, it can also trigger adverse allergic reactions.   And that is just one of the many synthetic additives in the processed foods and beverages that most people consume on a daily basis.   Compare this to consuming 1 cup of broccoli, which contains natural calcium, iron, magnesium, phosphorus, potassium, zinc, vitamin C, thiamin, riboflavin, niacin, vitamin B-6, folate, vitamin A, and more!   You are going to feel a huge difference in your energy and vitality when consuming nutrient dense foods of the same caloric value as processed foods. You may even see a pleasant shift on the bathroom scale as the body uses it or loses it - instead of storing these substances in our fat tissues through an inability to naturally eliminate them!

3. Plan out your menus: Shooting from the hip at 5:00 p.m. every evening about what to serve for dinner will only lead to massive doses of stress. In addition, when you finally settle on something, you may not even have the ingredients on-hand. I grew up in a household where both parents worked. I saw, from an early age, just how reliant my mother was on the pre-planned, weekly menus that she kept taped to the fridge. She shopped every Friday after school let out, armed with a list for the following week's menus. We spent many Saturday afternoons cooking and baking, and the freezer was permanently stocked. It was an invaluable lesson in being prepared, and ensuring that no matter the situation, a meal could always be heated in time for dinner.

4. Bulk cook: I bulk cook at least twice a week, making sure that I have staples like cooked whole grains, fish, poultry and steamed vegetables on-hand. I don't always plan a week of menus in advance, but I do try to go to bed at night having planned the following evening's dinner in my mind. I have been in the food business for many years though, and am a veteran of cooking fast, and in large quantities. If that is not you, then I suggest a little more foresight. Aim to bulk cook once or twice a week, yielding pieces of meals that can be rolled into other days of the week. You have to rely on your team here. If you are able to have an hour or two each week to shop while your partner or a respite caregiver is at home, you will have an opportunity to put this method into practice. If you cannot get out, have groceries delivered to your door. Many busy professionals employ this strategy. Below is a sample menu for a typical week in my home. You will notice how menu items are used multiple times, reducing the quantity of individual items I need to prepare overall each evening.

5. Be Prepared: I have yet to meet a mother who relishes the idea of getting up in the morning to make lunch boxes. I recommend tackling the arduous task at night after dinner. The beauty of this strategy is that you can use leftovers from dinner to make a great lunch platter or bento box. The greater goal is to prepare snacks and meals for yourself for the following day, and if dad gets a meal for work as a benefit, well that is just the icing on the cake! Once your day starts the following morning, we all know that every minute is going to be accounted for, so be prepared.

It is not all cooking. You need to fuel your body with a regular intake of high nutrient, good quality food. These can be in the form of snacks too. Pack your purse or a lunch hamper for your day. Have a bag specifically for the car filled with bottled water, snack bars, fresh fruit, tiny snack bags of pre-portioned nuts, rice cakes with yummy spreads, whatever it takes to keep your body fueled and your metabolism moving. The important thing is not to let hunger set in just as you arrive home from carpool or work. Your hunger will be a distraction from the myriad things needing to be accomplished over those next crucial hours. If you are irritable because your last meal was lunch five hours ago, you will not function optimally.

	BREAKFAST	LUNCH	DINNER
SUNDAY	Whole grain pancakes with toppings: berries, butter, Greek yogurt, maple syrup, nuts and seeds	Turkey sandwich or wrap with greens and tomato; Fresh fruit	4-5 oz Broiled salmon fillet, steamed seasonal veggies, wheat or gluten free pasta marinara
MONDAY	Protein shake; Oatmeal with toppings: berries, banana, seeds, maple syrup; Plain yogurt with fresh fruit and seeds	Leftover salmon wrap with tomato and greens; Fresh fruit	Cashew chicken and vegetable stir-fry over brown rice; Tossed salad
TUESDAY	Protein shake; Oatmeal with toppings: berries, banana, seeds, maple syrup; Plain yogurt with fresh fruit and seeds	Leftover stir-fry over sautéed kale; Fresh fruit	Vegetable and cheese stuffed shells marinara; Tossed or Caesar salad
WEDNESDAY	Protein shake; Oatmeal with toppings: berries, banana, seeds, maple syrup; Plain yogurt with fresh fruit and seeds	Leftover salmon and kasha pilaf; Tossed salad; Fresh fruit	Falafel with whole grain pita bar; Taco or fajita bar; Tossed salad
THURSDAY	Protein shake; Oatmeal with toppings: berries, banana, seeds, maple syrup; Plain yogurt with fresh fruit and seeds	Leftover falafel, fajita or taco salad; Fresh fruit	Soup and "make your own" Panini station

Acceptance — It's About The Journey

As the famous Ralph Waldo Emerson said, "Life is a journey, not a destination." For parents of special needs children that phrase is extremely resonant. A destination implies something finite, an end in and of itself to be strived for, like a miracle cure, or the mindset that if we throw enough time, money and intervention at our children all their struggles will fade away. It is a nice thought for about ten seconds! Then reality sets back in, and for most of us whose children have diagnoses that they will carry with them throughout their lives, we face the stark reality that we are on a journey that will last a lifetime. If and when our children grow up, master their challenges - and hopefully for some of them find something productive to do with their lives, as well as a partner to share it with - we will always be their parent and the worry will always nest in the depths of our soul.

Here's another newsflash: We are not perfect. Even when we think we are doing everything right, it still may not be good enough, and that is not necessarily our faults. As parents we cannot be expected to be experts at everything, but we can assume responsibility for having as much information at our fingertips as is possible (or affordable) to acquire. Sometimes we are in possession of the facts at the right moment in time and can prevent a calamity. More often than not, however, it has been my experience that we learn out of necessity, and in retrospect. While this is extremely frustrating in the moment, it is logical in that we cannot control everything that will happen and we cannot know the outcome until *after* it happens. If you do not want this to drive you completely crazy, you have to embrace the journey. You have to have the clarity to know that more craziness is coming right at you, and you are going to handle it because you are a seasoned traveler. You have a guide book that keeps growing, day in and day out. Whether you have the insight to acknowledge that fact, or even to write about it in your journal, or whether you appreciate in retrospect your instinctive and appropriate response when a situation arises, you will find over time that you are an expert in *many things special needs*. You may not be a doctor, a therapist, or a special education teacher, but you will have accumulated enough hands-on experience that will enable you to assist other parents on their journeys, and to be their tour guide.

Living in fear of the unknown is not an option. Sorry folks, it just isn't. When our children were younger, we would avoid certain situations in case one of them acted out inappropriately. Avoidance is like a band aid. It may be a temporary panacea, but in the long run, if you leave a wound untended it tends to fester -

and it certainly does not heal. As I grow older, I am less interested in what others think, and far more concerned with my own personal journey in search of optimal health, and with my children's progress. I don't fear failure; I don't fear lack of success; I don't fear imperfection; I don't even fear not reaching some ultimate destination of my imagining. The only thing I fear is inertia. Fear freezes, it undermines confidence, it mutes our inner voice, it clouds our judgment. When we allow fear to dominate us, we stall in our paths and the journey comes to a screeching halt.

How can we cultivate a positive view of our journey with our children? We can be flexible and patient. Nothing momentous is achieved overnight. Don't sweat the small stuff. Let non-essential tasks and activities slide. Continuously evaluate your battles on a sliding scale from "must deal with this immediately" to penciling it in for another day. Destinations can be the achievement of small goals, baby steps in the progression of our children's daily struggles to be less like their diagnosis and more like their peers. As my children entered their teen years, this was their singular goal. While it hurt me to see their determination to be more like everyone else and be dismissive of their own beautiful qualities, I had to constantly try and imagine what it must be like to walk in their shoes. How would I react to being bullied, or to being left off the guest list to a party, or to being the only person in the grade to not have a best friend, or sometimes any friend, or having to use a keyboard because I could not write, or being called a freak in the hallways? My children have experienced all of these situations and more.

The job will never be done, and the journey will continue, and that needs to be embraced. So, wake up each morning and behold the strength and beauty and wonder that are your children.

Conclusion:

Live, Learn, Love And Let Fly

"My mission in life is not merely to survive, but to thrive; and to do so with some passion, some compassion, some humor, and some style."
Maya Angelou

There are so many strategies one can employ to improve our health and well-being. After all is said and done though, we cannot lose sight of the fact that life passes us by in the blink of an eye. If we don't wake up each day with the intention of making every minute count, we will lose precious opportunities to live, to simply be present in the moment, to open ourselves to the myriad experiences that make life interesting and uniquely ours. It is never too late to learn something new, or to employ a new strategy. In fact, growing in knowledge and experience validates daily life. Challenges come and go, and fixating on them is akin to unlocking your door for the night thief and leaving him a glass of milk! In order to experience life with an endless flow of vitality, you have to play life forward, not react to it in a manner that propels you backwards. When I began my journey to take back control of my health, I felt overwhelmed and inadequate to the task at hand. I had to learn to accept that ten steps forward followed by five steps back was still indeed a net gain.

Release is a primary lesson on the adventure that is our lives. Releasing of stress, of situations, of relationships, of bad habits, and of our instinctive need to protect our children and determine their fates, is all vital to ensuring the quality of our physical and emotional health. Allowing children to make their own mistakes and to chart their own courses equates to forward momentum. If we constantly try and pre-empt their mistakes or carry a giant net on our shoulders in order to catch them as they fall, we are not serving them or ourselves well but only holding back progress. Let your babies fly, even if they come crashing down.

As someone who employees teenagers, it frightens me to witness the lack of common sense and the inability of young people today to problem-solve in the moment. There is also a deplorable lack of the skills necessary to be innovative. (Much of the blame rests with an educational system that has not kept pace with the needs of the twenty-first century.) The greatest gift we can give our children is, in a sense, a gift to ourselves too – giving them the space to develop these fundamental life skills through a cycle of failures and successes. And how much more important is this to the child with special challenges? Their lessons are doubly hard but critically more important.

Find elbow room in the world for yourself, and then widen the circle so you can move with more freedom and breathe a little more deeply. Live in a state of grace, knowing there is always someone worse off than you. So many parents I have had the privilege of interacting with shared the same heartfelt sentiment - gratitude for the cards they had been dealt. Throughout the pains and gains of their journeys, every one of them intuitively understood that, as hard as it was at times, there was always another parent and child out there with a challenge infinitely harder to overcome. From grace comes compassion, through compassion blossoms love. Shower yourself and your circle with unconditional love.

We have come full circle and end with the same premise as we started, that for all parents of a special needs children, juggling daily living is complex and challenging. With the scrutiny of a judiciary we constantly access whether or not we can shrug off the universal guilt we experience at concerning ourselves with ourselves.

I will leave you with a parting thought. A very wise sage once said:

"If I am not for myself, who will be for me? And if I am for myself, what am I? And if not now, when?"

Ethics of our Fathers, Chapter One.

Resources

Definitions of Alternative Health & Medical Practices

I make reference throughout the book to functional and integrative medicine. For the purposes of clarity, I want to give you a brief definition of what these practices encompass.

A. The Institute of Functional Medicine describes it as follows: "Functional medicine addresses the underlying causes of disease, using a systems-oriented approach and engaging both patient and practitioner in a therapeutic partnership. It is an evolution in the practice of medicine that better addresses the healthcare needs of the 21st century. By shifting the traditional disease-centered focus of medical practice to a more patient-centered approach, functional medicine addresses the whole person, not just an isolated set of symptoms. Functional medicine practitioners spend time with their patients, listening to their histories and looking at the interactions among genetic, environmental, and lifestyle factors that can influence long-term health and complex, chronic disease. In this way, functional medicine supports the unique expression of health and vitality for each individual." https://www.functionalmedicine.org

B. "Integrative medicine and health reaffirms the importance of the relationship between practitioner and patient, focuses on the whole person, is informed by evidence, and makes use of all appropriate therapeutic and lifestyle approaches, healthcare professionals and disciplines to achieve optimal health and healing." The Academic Consortium for Integrative Medicine and Health. https://www.imconsortium.org/about/about-us.cfm.

C. Naturopathic medicine uses natural methods to heal the body. These include herbs, vitamins and supplements, and holistic practices such as massage, exercising and dietary controls.

D. Homeopathic medicine treats the whole person as opposed to focusing on one of the body's systems. The American Institute of Homeopathy additionally describes three key principles in treatment focus: 1) Let Likes Cure Likes - a process whereby remedies are prescribed that most closely resonate with the characteristic of the patient's complaint; 2) The Minimum Dose – patients are prescribed the minimum dose necessary to effect a change, with the least amount of side effects; 3) The Single Remedy – only one remedy is prescribed at a time in order to evaluate the true effects, without these effects being compromised. http://homeopathyusa.org/homeopathic-medicine.html

E. Chiropractic medicine focusses on spinal alignment, and the alignment of the entire body's structure. Alignment, especially spinal alignment, is key to reducing points of pain and discomfort in the body in order to achieve optimal health. Chiropractors rely on spinal manipulation, heat treatment, electrical stimulation and lifestyle choices to promote recovery.

F. Physical therapy attempts to correct or alleviate symptoms that restrict physical movement, and the pain and discomfort associated with the affliction. Physical therapy relies on massage, heat treatments, exercises, diet and lifestyle accommodations for rehabilitation.

FOOD IDEAS:

Lunch Boxes

Following are some links to some of my favorite lunch box systems, and Target now stocks lunch boxes that have bento-style interiors and which are much more affordable.

https://www.theultimategreenstore.com/m-29-laptop-lunches-bentology.aspx

https://bentology.com

Bento Box Lunch Ideas

- Apple and nut butter sandwiches (no bread)
- String cheese and cottage cheese
- Frozen peas and corn combo
- Pumpkin, apple, banana, blueberry, zucchini, or corn muffins
- Popcorn
- Fruit slices, salad, purees, and sauces
- Hard boiled or devilled eggs
- Caprese salad of mozzarella balls or cubes, baby tomatoes and pesto
- Trail mixes – store bought or home-made
- Granola, plain yogurt and fresh fruit cubes

- Home-made soups
- Whole wheat pancake sandwiches
- Hummus and veggie sticks
- Guacamole and/or salsa with tortilla chips
- Lara Bars
- Kind Bars
- Whole wheat pasta marinara
- Whole grain salads of quinoa, wheatberries, brown and wild rice, cous cous
- Pita pockets with veggies, cheeses, and spreads
- Wraps
- Tuna salad and tuna pasta salad
- Quesadillas filled with sliced veggies, refried beans, cheese, guacamole, tuna, etc.
- Falafel with techina dipping sauce, or in half a pita with salad
- Mini muffin quiches
- Frittata slices
- Apple or corn fritters

Green Smoothie Recipes For Energy And Vitality

"Appley Ever After" Smoothie

2 Cups Baby Kale, Spinach or Mixed Greens
1 Cup Water
½ Cup Nut, Rice or Coconut Milk
1 Green Apple Diced (Skin and Pits Included)
½ Banana
¼ Avocado
1-2 Pitted Dates
1 Serving Protein Powder of Your Choice
1 Tbsp Chia Seeds
1 Tbsp Ground Flax Seed

Island Dream Smoothie

2 Cups Kale of your Choice
1 Cup Coconut Milk, Coconut Water or Plain Water
1 Cup Frozen Tropical Fruit of Your Choice: Banana, Papaya,
Pineapple, Mango, Passionfruit Pulp, Guava
1 Tbsp Coconut Butter
1 Tbsp Chia Seeds
1 Tbsp Ground Flax Seeds
1 Serving Vanilla Protein Powder

Choco Monkey Smoothie

1 Cup Kale, Spinach or Mixed Greens
1 Cup Almond, Rice or Hemp Milk
½ Avocado
1 Banana
1 Tbsp Cocoa Powder
1 Serving Chocolate Protein Powder
2 Tbsp Ground Flax Seeds

Acid Versus Alkaline Foods

ALKALINE	ACID
Veggies - Leafy greens	Meat/Dairy
Whole grains	Refined/Processed Foods
Fruit	Sugar
Water	Drugs/Alcohol
Lemon, Apple Cider Vinegar	Coffee
Green/Herbal Tea	Soda

"Dirty Dozen" Produce List

(Courtesy of the Environmental Working Group.)

Buy only organic when possible

1. Strawberries
2. Apples
3. Nectarines
4. Peaches
5. Celery
6. Grapes
7. Cherries
8. Spinach
9. Tomatoes
10. Bell Peppers
11. Cherry Tomatoes
12. Cucumber

LOW MERCURY FISH

LEAST MERCURY:
Anchovies
Butterfish
Catfish
Clam
Crab (Domestic)
Crawfish/Crayfish
Croaker (Atlantic)
Flounder
Hake
Herring
Jacksmelt (Silverside)
Mackerel (N. Atlantic Chub)
Mullet
Oyster
Plaice
Pollock
Salmon (Canned)
Salmon (Fresh)
Sardine
Scallop
Shrimp
Sole (Pacific)
Squid (Calamari)
Tilapia
Whitefish
Whiting

MODERATE MERCURY:
(Consume 6 or less servings per month)
Bass (Striped, Black)
Buffalofish
Carp

Cod (Alaskan)
Lobster
Mahi Mahi
Monkfish
Perch (Freshwater)
Sheepshead
Skate
Snapper
Tilefish (Atlantic)
Tuna (canned chunk light, skipjack)

HIGH MERCURY:
(Consume 3 or less servings per month)
Croaker (White Pacific)
Halibut (Atlantic & Pacific)
Mackerel (Spanish, Gulf)
Perch (Ocean)
Sable Fish
Sea Bass (Chilean)
Tuna (Albacore, yellowfin)

HIGHEST MERCURY:
(Avoid Eating)
Bluefish
Grouper
Mackerel (King)
Marlin
Orange Roughy
Shark
Swordfish
Tuna (Bigeye, Ahi)

(Source: The Natural Resources Defense Council at www.nrdc.org)

Acknowledgements

There is simply no way I would have managed this journey without the help of my immediate family members, to whom I am forever indebted. Aside from their infinite love, support and understanding, I am so grateful to you for the following:

My parents, Delia and Bobby. You provided countless hours, days and nights of respite. Mom, as a life-long educator, you really understood the importance of meeting each individual child's needs. Your years of expertise kept us calm as you helped handle the children. Dad, I'm glad you did not have a heart attack in the process of babysitting!! You have the patience of a saint! Thanks for all the carpools, grocery runs, doctor appointment runs, and so much more. Thanks for also having my back at work.

My in-laws, Rene and David. Not a day went by in California when there was not a grandparent in our house lending a hand, and you sure put in your hours. Mum, you know that I actually did, and still do, listen to you. You are not "just" the mother-in-law. You provide sage counsel and force me be to be a realist about my expectations of being a "Superwoman". And Dad, your help with money matters and investment advice helped me create sound financial practices.

My brother, Arnie, himself an author: You started me off on my journey to health, and for that I am forever grateful. You have a way of making us all see ourselves in the mirror, and it is an awakening experience. You have been an inspirational and creative force in our home.

My sister, Justine: No matter how crazy life was, or how many insane antics my children got up to, you would come over and be funny and bring your bubbly laughter into our home and infuse us all. You are a safe space for my children and I am most grateful for that!

So many others have been there for us in so many important ways. To my husband's siblings, all the sibling's spouses, our nieces and nephews, our aunts and uncles, you have been the village.

Our friends have become like our family. We have shared the laughter, the pain, the tears, advice, resources, meals, babysitting and so much more. We are woven into the fabric of each other's lives. Thank you Mel and Steve, Lauren and Derek, Dan and Diane, Jodi and Col, Barry and Judy for being our rocks!

To Joshua Rosenthal, you have created a movement that is going to change the world and I feel privileged to be part of it. Dr. Mark Hyman, Dr. Todd LePine and the wonderful, caring staff at The UltraWellness Center. You have given me the gift of understanding who I am physically, and how I can coach my body into being vibrant and healthy for many years to come.

About The Author

Lara Franks is a Certified Health Coach and a graduate of the Institute for Integrative Nutrition. She is the founder of Frankly Healthier Living, a wellness company focusing on coaching clients to optimal health through dietary and lifestyle changes.

Lara has been in the food industry for over 25 years and is a health food chef. She is a partner in a food services company that owns and operates three restaurants and a division that provides meals to educational institutions, as well as specially formulated patient meals to hospitals and weight loss clients.

Hailing from South Africa, where she graduated with a degree in education, Lara emigrated to the United States in 1991. She is married with four children and three dogs.